Sleep

A Comprehensive Guide to Improving Physical

(Practical Knowledge to Sleep Better and Improve Your Life)

Marshall Green

Published By **John Kembrey**

Marshall Green

Sleep: A Comprehensive Guide to Improving Physical (Practical Knowledge to Sleep Better and Improve Your Life)

ISBN   978-1-998927-04-3

Legal & Disclaimer

Upon using the information contained in this book, you agree to hold harmless the Author from and against any damages, costs, and expenses, including any legal fees potentially resulting from the application of any of the information provided by this guide. This disclaimer applies to any damages or injury caused by the use and application, whether directly or indirectly, of any advice or information presented, whether for breach of contract, tort, negligence, personal injury, criminal intent, or under any other cause of action.

You agree to accept all risks of using the information presented inside this book. You need to consult a professional medical practitioner in order to ensure you are both able and healthy enough to participate in this program.

Table Of Contents

Chapter 1: Understanding Sleep

Sleep is a physiological country of self-law and rest. It stays one of the maximum mysterious abilties of the human thoughts, and in spite of the truth that we spend a third of our lives asleep, we recognise very little about it.

Until currently, it come to be notion that when we asleep the mind is at relaxation, inactive, however thanks to advances in era and with the primary statistics of the encephalogram, we located out that the thoughts is some distance from inactive in the route of this time.

In truth, it's miles without a doubt the opportunity; the thoughts is intensively energetic on the identical time as we're asleep. So what takes place at the same time as we sleep? What is the circadian rhythm? What are sleep degrees and the way do they have an effect on us? Keep analyzing, we're quite a whole lot to start.

Importance Of Biorhythms (Inner Clock)

Our lifestyles is based virtually in a twenty-four hour rhythm, equal to the trade of moderate and darkness provoked via the earth's rotation around the solar. Many techniques in our body present the same rhythmical direction in a length of twenty-4 hours; it's what we name biorhythm. Biorhythm and most of those techniques are regulated through a organic clock. This inner clock that governs every person is positioned in the center of the mind, tiny cells with a curly shape.

You see, this lifestyles clock, which each person have, works in a twenty-four hour layout, as to say it repeats every twenty-four hours. It's our cycle of interest and relaxation, that is why we every now and then revel in active and some different times we genuinely experience tired and sleepy.

Many organic features in humans, which incorporates the intervals of wakefulness and sleep, hormonal interest, and body temperature are set up in a natural way:

constant with a circadian rhythm that develops along a cycle of approximately sooner or later.

The circadian rhythm uses the mild of the day to synchronize human beings with their surroundings. In mornings, multiple hours earlier than you awaken, the circadian rhythm makes your body produce large quantities of cortisol, referred to as the "pressure hormone," to put together you for the day. Also, blood pressure will growth and sugar is released to your blood so that you will be active and alert at some point of the day. In distinct phrases, it turns on you so that you can paintings and stay. This identical circadian rhythm augments the melatonin ranges in your body at night time time. Melatonin is a hormone that relaxes you and diminishes essential abilities so that you can sleep and rest.

The circadian rhythm adjustments with time and age because teenagers and teens sleep extra. Older humans will be inclined to sleep earlier and arise earlier, but as we age we additionally typically generally tend to sleep masses a great deal much less, and this is actually regular. But every so often our organic clock is altered for brilliant instances, inner or outdoor, and a discrepancy is produced inside the circadian rhythm. When this occurs, the obligations and skills of the frame waft at a unique rhythm; we aren't programmed for this.

When the natural rhythm of someone advances or receives no longer on time artificially, the internal organic rhythms (as the wakefulness and sleep rhythm) don't readjust with out difficulty or rapid. This lack of synchronization can produce many bodily discomforts and disorientation that would very last days or even weeks.

It's crucial to be aware about this inner clock we have were given; we can't forget about the herbal rhythms of our frame. Factories, machines, and electric facilities artwork continuously at some point of twenty-four hours: day and night time time, non-prevent. Cars, automobiles, planes, and ships supply merchandise around the world clearly in time, but the human frame can't look at this rhythm; we need to relaxation, in unique phrases, we want to sleep.

The human frame is a super and smart device, and there's a logical purpose for us spending a 3rd a part of our life sound asleep. Even even though we aren't privy to some thing at the equal time as we're asleep, in the course of this era of time many important skills which can be vital for staying healthy rise up in our frame. Sleeping properly at night time may be the difference among burning fats or preserving it, amongst been healthy or lousy, and take delivery of as actual with it or now not, among dwelling a long healthful existence or a hastily declining one.

There are one million hypotheses about the features of sleep, but among all those viable abilties, we have were given the perfect diploma of scientifically showed evidence about the following few.

•Recovery of chemical power inside the body

•Memorization and consolidation of what we've discovered out in the end of wakefulness

•Regulation of mind's temperature

•Elimination of the pollutants the mind produces at the same time as we are wakeful

•Repair of body tissue

•Cerebral plasticity

How Many Hours Of Sleep?

This varies in step with age, however it is able to moreover range in folks who are the identical age. Babics can sleep round seventeen hours a day, and then the ones hours are decreased to ten and 9 hours as they expand.

The majority of adults want among seven and eight hours every night time, even though as we grow older this time can lessen. What is in truth vital is how many sleep cycles you complete. Several research have confirmed that the quantity of hours you sleep don't determine how rested you sense tomorrow.

So, because of this that someone that sleeps masses of hours doesn't constantly will revel in fresh and wonderful the following morning. Is this statistics to you? Don't worry we'll get into that.

Stages Of Sleep

Your body, or your mind to be extra precise, goes via a series of severa tiers while you sleep. It's important you comprehend a touch approximately those because of the truth, as I advised you earlier than, they have masses to do with how masses we in reality rest and the way suitable we'll experience in the course of the morning. So allow's get into it.

Stage I

Somnolence; moreover called slight sleep. Just as you close up your eyes and nod off the brain enters the number one diploma. This first degree is just like the middle zone between been asleep and big huge conscious. You come and exit of sleep and can be easily woke up. During this stage muscular tension is reduced, the eyes flow into very slowly, and breathing slows down.

Stage II

Superficial sleep: the movement of the eyes stops; the waves of the mind increase, slow down, and are normal. All the senses are blocked, however this doesn't recommend that sleep at some point of this level is repairing. We're no longer there however, simply a bit greater.

Stage III

Slightly deep sleep: thoughts waves growth in period and slowness. The competencies of the complete organism are slower and slower every time. These gradual waves are known as delta waves, and that they change with smaller and faster waves. If someone wakes you up within the route of this degree of sleep, you can experience disoriented.

Stage IV

Deep sleep: cutting-edge unconsciousness, pretty lengthy, soft, and sluggish mind waves. During this degree of deeper sleep, the thoughts produces almost definitely delta waves and is even as the organism recuperates bodily and mentally. There's no ocular motion or muscle interest. In the case there are goals in this level they wouldn't be like a movie as they generally are, however with shapes and lighting fixtures, quite psychedelic.

Stage V

As someone gradually goes thru the ranges of sleep the mind styles draw slow waves, but whilst we beautify into the V level something top notch takes region: the REM sleep, or rapid eye movement sleep, it really is the fifth and very last degree of sleep. The REM sleep is so particular that the rest of the stages are certainly called Non-REM degrees. This diploma is so terrific due to the fact the thoughts is not drawing slow waves anymore, however chaotic lines that advise you're wide unsleeping, however you really are asleep. This degree is characterized with the aid of speedy eye movements and is discovered through colourful goals, rich in content material, hues, and sensations. During REM, the blood go together with the glide to the thoughts accelerates, and breathing is faster, the brain stops emitting signs to the bone marrow, and your muscle tissues are nonetheless, which impedes you shifting like crazy and performing your dreams.

Sleep Cycle

After ten minutes in the REM diploma, you descend to the Non-REM ranges, and you will be going from the Non-REM to the REM stages for the duration of the complete night time time. A wholesome person will spend about 5% of the sleeping time in degree 1; 25% in stage 2; 45% in tiers 3 and four; and

25% inside the REM degree. The whole cycle of REM and Non-REM lasts approximately amongst ninety to 100 twenty mins, so 8 hours of sleep may additionally additionally have 4 or 5 cycles.

Doing Some Math!

Your brain and your body want to complete an entire cycle; waking up inside the middle of the personal, and most profound sleep isn't always appropriate in any respect. Considering that a whole sleep cycle is of about ninety minutes, is it better to set the alarm after 3 hours of sleep, or 4.Five hours, or 6 six hours, or 7.Five hours, or nine hours? Hmmm…In theory the answer is sure; in reality every person is first-rate. The ninety mins is not a rule, it is able to range from ninety mins to one hundred and twenty minutes. Besides, expertise the proper time you go to sleep and setting your alarm consistent with that may be tough. But, there are some devices that may do that for you, and when you have problem waking up within the morning, this may be a first rate solution.

Now to complete this chapter, I'll like to go through some of the outstanding advantages an fantastic night time time sleep can provide you with. Sleeping well way you experience properly widespread fitness. Despite the frenetic rhythm of life in recent times, sleep is a easy necessity that shouldn't be unnoticed. Sleep brings loads of advantages for your health and thoughts. Let's go through some of the ones.

Benefits Of Sleeping Properly

The following are some key blessings of having an extremely good nights rest:

Sleep maintains your heart healthful: coronary heart assaults are more frequent at a few stage in the first hours of the morning, and this will be explained with the way sleep interacts along side your blood vessels.

Sleep improves your reminiscence: as , your mind is exquisite energetic even as you're at asleep. During this time, your reminiscence consolidates everything you located whilst you have got been aware.

Sleep diminishes strain: stress and sleep have an impact on your cardiovascular health. Sleep reduces your stages of strain and so that you manage your blood stress higher.

Sleep controls urge for meals: whilst you sleep properly your frame regulates the hormones that produce starvation. Keeping your hormones in take a look at with an exceptional night time sleep can be very beneficial.

Sleep protection your frame: your frame produces more protein molecules at the same time as you sleep, and those improve your ability to combat infections and hold you wholesome. These molecules assist your body heal on a cell diploma while you are pressured or you are exposed to dangerous elements or bacteria.

Sleep helps in interest and recognition: many researchers take into account that even as you sleep your neurons can save you and join the harm that came about all through the day.

Sleep enables with melancholy: sleep has a excellent impact on many chemical materials for your body, alongside facet serotonin. A pinnacle night time time time's sleep helps your thoughts release the ones chemical materials and be happier.

Sleep upkeep tissue: hormone manufacturing is regularized at some point of sleep. Also, the tissue is repaired in your organism at the same time as you sleep, which incorporates corrections within the harm because of UV moderate inside the pores and pores and skin. A applicable night time time's sleep will repair your skin and your body.

Sleep permits you stay longer: this is why sleep is related to such a variety of fitness benefits. If you've got a healthy body, you have got a healthy life and live longer.

Sleep improves creativity: except enhancing and strengthening reminiscence, your brain reorganizes your reminiscences, and this translates into extra creativity. While you sleep the emotional components of a memory are strengthened, and this enables inside the revolutionary manner.

Chapter 2: Health Implications Of Improper Sleep

Daily life sports can now and again make people forget approximately the importance of a terrific night time time's sleep and right rest. The fact is, each dwelling being with a worried gadget desires to sleep, and we are not an exception. Several research suggest that those who sleep a whole lot a good deal much less than six hours every night time are at greater hazard of loss of life, and tremendous after one night time of now not sound asleep properly cerebral tissue is lost.

So, you get the photograph now? A correct night time's sleep isn't only vital; it is critical. Let's go through some of the horrible consequences of now not dozing properly or no longer slumbering enough.

Effects Of Not Sleeping

Hunger and tension: loss of sleep provokes a unethical to ingest greater electricity, carbohydrates, and is associated with junk meals cravings.

Increases twist of fate risk: that is in fact a no brainer, it's examined that individuals who don't sleep properly are at greater threat of been involved in a automobile twist of fate. The ocular coordination outcomes are those that play an vital element in this.

Less appealing: luggage below the eyes, worn-out appearance and untimely pores and skin growing older are some of the outcomes of no longer slumbering well. The hormone that offers elasticity to the pores and pores and skin and prevents wrinkles is released at some stage in the night time, so sleep has lots to do with you getting dates, or now not getting any.

More possibilities to get the flu: safety mechanisms to your frame are affected by the dearth of sleep.

Loss of cerebral tissue: this is due to how the mind overloads with the dearth of sleep affecting the fearful machine.

Overly emotional: sleep, feelings, and behaviors percent a complicated blend of chemical substances in the mind, so the lack of sleep makes your thoughts paintings more hard and the apprehensive system is affected by this.

Memory problems: tiredness does now not permit the thoughts to manner records effectively, and this accumulates throughout the whole day. The mind is incapable of maintaining facts and memory is not precise.

Difficulty focusing and concentrating: tiredness and sleepiness keep away from absolutely everyone searching for to recognition; this is straightforward. The thoughts doesn't get sufficient blood and it is able to't function at a excessive diploma.

Augments threat of embolism: the dearth of sleep can located your frame in a steady country of alert, and this augments the manufacturing of hormones that reason strain and anxiety, scary an boom for your blood strain.

Increases threat of suffering from weight issues: this is additionally due to hormones, like ghrelin and leptin, which paintings in opposition to you even as you don't get sufficient sleep. Here's a great ebook in leptin resistance

Increases threat of laid low with most cancers: numerous research accomplice the shortage of sleep with colon and breast maximum cancers.

Diabetes: the frame's response to now not dozing is similar to what takes vicinity even as diabetes is really starting. When there's insulin resistance the sugar ranges inside the frame increase and reason organ failure.

Cardiac problems: lack of sleep elevates blood strain and this can provoke artery obstruction and cardiac failure.

Affects fertility: a whole lot much less focus of sperm within the semen is what provokes this.

Lack of sleep affects genes: interruption of sleep or loss of sleep influences extra than seven hundred genes, and for this the chance of suffering from illnesses like maximum cancers, diabetes, and masses of others growth.

Lack of sleep is likewise associated with anxiety, depression, diminution of libido, mood swings, terrible mood, and the propensity of many chronic illnesses. Now which you understand all that could seem in case you don't relaxation well I bet you'll pay extra hobby to your biological clock and the wishes of your frame.

Sleeping Disorders

Sleep is like a trademark of your health in standard. Healthy human beings generally tend to sleep nicely, however when you have slumbering issues, this will be a trademark of an underlying hassle. There are many things together with strain, caffeine, cigarettes, loss of exercise, and plenty of others. That can reason sleeping troubles. But in case you often have problem snoozing at night time time, then maybe there's something else. We'll communicate a number of the maximum common snoozing problems so you can check in case you is probably coping with a drowsing problem.

Insomnia

Insomnia is one of the most not unusual snoozing issues. Many humans complain they don't sleep enough or that their sleep modified into surely now not incredible. This may be because of many things similar to the bed not being snug, noises, immoderate temperature, uncommon exercises, lack of bodily exercising, eating too much earlier than you go to mattress, alcohol, cigarettes, or caffeine liquids which incorporates coffee and tea. However, this occasionally may be due to emotional troubles, troubles in each day life, pressure, and depression.

Insomnia Symptoms

•Difficulty falling asleep

•Waking up inside the nighttime and being no longer capable of fall again asleep yet again

•Waking up several instances within the route of the night time time time

•Sleepiness and tiredness at a few degree within the day

Sleep Apnea

Sleep apnea is likewise a commonplace sleeping disease. Apnea takes location on the same time as your breathing stops momentarily sooner or later of sleep due to the reality your higher airways get blocked. This interrupts your respiration, and so your sleep additionally receives interrupted numerous instances in some unspecified time in the future of the night time time time. You won't don't forget the ones episodes, however the next day you may experience very tired. Sleep apnea may be mild or pretty intense, and it may be because of being overweight, pillows, a mild mattress, among special topics.

Sleep Apnea Symptoms

•Loud loud night breathing, normally persistent

•Pauses in breathing in the direction of sleep

•Choking, panting, hassle respiratory in the course of sleep

•Feeling tired and without power at some stage in the day even after snoozing for prolonged hours

•Waking up with headaches, dry throat, nasal congestion, or chest pain

Restless Leg Syndrome

Restless Leg Syndrome reasons an impossible to resist preference to transport the legs. People who be with the aid of this syndrome experience uncomfortable while they are in bed. Some human beings describe it as a tingling, crawling sensation. As with one-of-a-kind drowsing problems, alcohol, caffeine, and cigarettes can get worse the symptoms.

Advanced Sleep Phase Syndrome

Advanced Sleep Phase Syndrome is even as human beings aren't capable of live wakeful during instances in which they'll be supposed to be lively, really in order that they sleep brief and early, however awaken in the middle of the night and might't fall back asleep. This syndrome is extra common amongst older people.

Delayed Sleep Phase Syndrome

Delayed Sleep Phase Syndrome is a lot more commonplace than Advanced Sleep Phase Syndrome, defined above. It's characterized thru trouble sound asleep. People who be affected by manner of this syndrome sleep later than everyday and feature problem waking up within the morning. This can cause immoderate issues due to the truth these human beings's greater lively hours are beyond midnight. This can purpose troubles in paintings, university, or morning sports. This syndrome develops mainly some of the some time of sixteen and 18, similarly to at some stage in the twenties. It's extremely good to look it increase within the thirties or later in existence.

Nightmares

Nightmares are common, and I dare to mention that everybody has suffered from nightmares at the least as soon as of their lifetime. But, what isn't always not unusual is to be concerned with the resource of nightmares every day. Food, strain, or emotional issues can unchain those terrible night time research.

Bruxism

Bruxism is a sleep trouble that appears within the 2nd diploma of sleep and is characterized with the beneficial aid of lateral mandibular movements that reason intense friction many of the top and decrease tooth. It's nocturnal tooth grinding, and it could provoke extreme tooth damage and facial ache.

Any of these slumbering issues, because of pressure or adjustments in the circadian rhythm can initiate tiredness, irritability, digestive upsets, and one-of-a-kind symptoms and signs that may be worrying and in reality traumatic. There are many things you may do to help your frame sleep higher and deliver your brain and your frame a few relaxation. If the problems persist, please visit your physician.

Chapter 3: Diet & Sleep

As you understand, sleep deprivation should have extreme dangerous consequences for your famous health, so supporting your body get a amazing night time sleep isn't always this type of awful idea. How are you able to try this? The first detail you want is to be aware that now not most effective pressure and problems have an effect on your sleep, but your diet additionally plays an important feature in all of this.

If you need to sleep like a infant, if you want to keep away from waking up inside the middle of the night or having hassle drowsing, you have to comprehend and take shipping of that what you eat at some point of the day, in particular within the previous couple of hours in advance than snoozing, affects you.

The food you consume for dinner or inside the hours before you doze off has a excellent effect in your sleep. Food should have an effect at the first-class and length of your sleep. This is why it's so critical to eat healthful, particularly at dinnertime; eating food that paintings together together together with your frame and now not against it. If you assist your self with the proper substances, I can assure you, you may sleep higher each night time time, and with the useful resource of doing this you may sense well, extra lively and rested each day.

There's an instantaneous relation among your consuming behavior and sleep, this is due to the fact a few vitamins interact with hormones and chemical substances that have an impact for your rest and sleep. You see, hormones are answerable for wakefulness and sleep, and each states are associated with the circadian rhythm. This circadian rhythm can be altered, in particular after thirty years of age, thru stress, night time time shifts, prolonged intercontinental flights or your healthy eating plan. Luckily, there's masses you can do to assist your frame, and all of it starts offevolved with a right food plan.

Many people say that to have a awesome sleep, considerable and heavy dinners should be averted. This is without a doubt authentic, but it's also actual that you may't go to the opportunity excessive. You should in no way visit bed on an empty belly, or consuming so little which you wake up in the midnight along side your belly growling due to the fact you're ravenous. The ideal is to have a dinner that produces the sensation of satiety however primarily based in nonfat substances and of clean digestion.

It's additionally no longer recommendable to devour dinner and right away go to mattress; that is related to accumulation of fat and it does now not assist in sleep the least bit. The superb is to have dinner and wait an hour and 1/2 or hours before going to bed.

Hormones

Let's talk a touch approximately serotonin and melatonin; the ones are chemical substances that play such an crucial characteristic in sleep balance.

Serotonin is a neurotransmitter that actions records via unique components of your brain. It right away or circuitously controls almost every function of your mind, like your mood, sexual functions and sleep cycles. Serotonin tiers in your body are high at the same time as you are big wakeful and lively, and almost absent while you are in the private degree of sleep.

While you're asleep, melatonin degrees in your frame increase extensively. Melatonin production is based totally upon at the pineal gland, that is fed by using way of serotonin. While slight augments tiers of serotonin, darkness stimulates the producing of melatonin. For this cause, the proper quantities of serotonin and melatonin want to be decided to your frame to get an super and profound sleep.

Hormones And Diet

The release of those neurotransmitters is based totally upon at the availability of an amino acid known as tryptophan. Despite being an essential substance, tryptophan isn't produced manifestly in the body. Luckily, this amino acid is determined in plenty of meals that can assist stability the tiers of serotonin and melatonin that proper away have an impact for your sleep.

Foods High In Tryptophan

•Fish, specifically blue fish like sardines, mackerel and tuna. Also white fish like cod and halibut.

•Red meat

•Eggs

•Dairy merchandise as cheese and yogurt

•Legumes which includes lentil, chickpeas, peas, beans and peanuts

•Grains which incorporates rice, wheat, oatmeal and corn

•Dry culmination inclusive of almonds, pine nuts, pistachio and cashews

•Fruits like avocado, orange, dates, blueberries, grapes, apples, strawberries and cherries

•Vegetables which consist of spinach, zucchini, asparagus, celery, lettuce, tomatoes, carrots, cucumber and watercress

Other Important Nutrients

For the best enough release of those substances, besides tryptophan, Omega 3 and Omega 6 fatty acids are wished. You can discover those fatty acids in some fish like sardines, salmon, halibut, and cod or in dry fruits, olive and sunflower oil.

Magnesium is considered with the aid of the usage of many to be the "anti-pressure mineral," and they might be right. Low degrees of magnesium can cause slumbering troubles or symptoms and signs and symptoms and symptoms that interrupt your sleep. Augmenting your levels of magnesium will allow you to sleep higher at night time time as properly. Nuts, spinach, carrots and peas are wealthy in magnesium and Vitamin B6, which enables the metabolism of tryptophan. Bananas are like herbal sound asleep capsules, an injection of serotonin and melatonin and wealthy in magnesium: a natural muscle relaxer.

Calcium permits the mind make use of tryptophan more successfully, so melatonin is produced faster, and this induces sleep and rest. A small glass of heat milk also can assist plenty for a high-quality night's sleep in addition to yogurt.

Some carbs with low glycemic index additionally let you sleep. Glucose ranges within the blood inhibit hypocretin, that is a neurotransmitter that keeps you aware. But, don't forget, diploma is the essential difficulty. If you have got got a huge plate of pasta then the impact is probably the exact opposite; your digestion can be gradual and your sleep fragmented and no longer repairing in any respect. Oatmeal is one of the nice assets of melatonin, so keep it on your weight loss plan.

Vitamin C, positioned in oranges and kiwis, assist the frame hold the levels of magnesium energetic and interfere with the GABA, that is a neurotransmitter that inhibits the imperative worried device and is crucial for a excellent night time sleep.

An example of an awesome dinner is probably an omelet with zucchini or any vegetables you want, bird soup or vegetable soup, and a small a part of rice. A plate of salad with tomato, tuna and olive oil are also great alternatives for dinner. Oatmeal and blueberries, a heat glass of milk and some stop result can also assist. Use your creativeness; you have got lots of things to choose out from which can be healthy and will help you sleep like a little one!

What To Avoid

An excessive amount of meals for dinner, whether or not it includes tryptophan or now not, is honestly no longer beneficial for sleep. There are some assets you should clearly stay some distance from; permit's take a look at them out.

•Foods excessive in fats: these nutrients are the maximum hard to digest, so your stomach will even though art work whilst you are asleep. Fats make you feel heavy and they will be the primary element to avoid.

•Sugar: chocolate and sweets put off somnolence and make you alert, so please live far from them!

•Caffeine drinks which include espresso and tea must be avoided because of the fact they'll be stimulants. If you like espresso drink it at the least four or five hours earlier than you visit mattress. Now, sodas...overlook about approximately them. They are times worse in your sleep because of the reality they comprise caffeine and sugar.

•A glass of wine can be relaxing for loads, however even though it has a sedative impact, it does no longer produce a repairing sleep. Alcohol dehydrates your body and intervenes with the repairing effects of sleep.

•-Avoid ingesting liquids in excessive portions in advance than you sleep because it will make you arise to move the rest room at some point of the night time. Stay hydrated for the duration of the day, however keep liquids in check at night time time time.

These are the fundamentals of nutrients and sleep. Try to paintings collectively along with your frame; you will sense the difference. And remember that an tremendous night time's sleep will not satisfactory make you sense glowing and lively every day, however also prolong your existence and your amazing of life.

Chapter 4: Lifestyle & Sleep

A healthful manner of existence does no longer handiest affect your cutting-edge health, however moreover favors your sleep. Several studies mean that people who make well lifestyle choices experience correct health and sleep more profoundly.

There are behavior that have terrific results in every diploma of your sleep. Many of these behavior or life-style alternatives, which includes food plan, surroundings, and so forth. Are a rely extensive variety of commonplace revel in, however many humans usually usually tend to miss them and, as a result, be afflicted by insomnia or specific sound asleep issues.

Let's undergo some of those conduct that assist you to easy up your sleep, and please don't forget which you need to be consistent to get outstanding results.

Alcohol And Stimulants

You ought to be in reality careful with the ingestion of stimulants. Caffeine is a brilliant example: you may have a cup or at some stage in the day, however in case you drink many cups your sleep may be affected.

Nicotine is a stimulant drug that still interferes collectively with your sleep. Symptoms of night time time privation can interrupt your most first-class goals. Besides, cigarettes are virtually horrific for you!

Alcohol acts in a completely exceptional way in your body: at the begin it induces sleep, but then it's going to interrupt it. Only one cup can translate into waking up normally throughout the night time and nightmares. If you could drink, try and do it as a minimum four or 5 hours earlier than you go to bed, in reality as with espresso.

Exercise

Exercise no longer excellent allows your preferred health, but is important to get a incredible night time time sleep. This is a few thing you need to encompass on your every day ordinary.

Even even though workout is beneficial on your health and your sleep, the time of the day you discern out is important. People which may be in a incredible physical country need to keep away from exercising as a minimum six hours earlier than going to mattress.

Exercising within the morning will gain your sleep, however exercising in the afternoon or at a time that's close to your bedtime, can reason adjustments for your sleep. A sedentary lifestyles, abnormal or restricted bodily interest also can initiate insomnia or sleep disturbances. So get it shifting and schooling consultation a bit!

Stress Management

Stress is one of the most common matters that trigger insomnia, and there's a logical cause for this. When your body is underneath stress, your mind responds, activating your anxious device, and at the same time as this takes region your breathing and heart rate accelerate and your muscle tissues collect huge amounts of oxygen. As you may don't forget, with all this happening indoors you, sleep can grow to be mission not feasible. It's essential you discover ways to manipulate pressure and the way to preserve calm an superb manner to rest properly every night time time. In the following chapter we'll undergo some strategies that will help you loosen up and art work in your stress levels.

Night Routines

To experience brilliant sleep which could fulfill its reason and recharge your batteries, a night time time time regular that induces relaxation and sleep is vital.

For example, putting a schedule to visit mattress each night time is beneficial. Your body receives used to schedules, this shows you can get used to slumbering at the identical time every night time.

A right everyday may be having a healthful dinner, then a chilled shower, and on the identical time as you do this, disconnect your self from paintings and everything else. Then placed on snug garments, study a ebook and go to mattress and sleep like a toddler. Do this each day, precisely the identical manner and within the identical time table, your body gets used to it and your sleep will beautify genuinely.

Weight

If you have a few more pounds, attempt to eliminate them. Being overweight can reason sleep apnea and interruptions in your sleep.

Sleeping Pills

I would really like to finish this bankruptcy thru supplying you with a few information approximately sound asleep pills. Many people are determined, however aren't virtually aware of the outcomes and consequences.

Sleeping capsules had been used for a long term to assist folks who be through insomnia and other snoozing issues. In truth, we comprehend that capsules aren't the solution. They are poisonous and may initiate many severe aspect effects. In one-of-a-type terms, they'll be able to make you revel in miserable. Sleeping tablets can cause tiredness, irritability, and that they lose their effectiveness quite quick, because of this you could should augment the dose on every occasion, and that is risky. There are many stuff you could attempt in advance than the use of dozing tablets, so that you want to go away the ones at the problem.

Lifestyle impacts your sleep masses! Good way of existence alternatives are beneficial in your whole frame, not only your sleep. Be clever about what you do, what you consume and live wholesome in each element of your life.

Chapter 5: Five Miracle Exercises

Before we get into the miracle sports that will help you sleep better than you have got ever slept on your existence, permit's go through some subjects you want to cover first.

Preparing Your Bedroom

If you're analyzing this, it technique you have got already were given made modifications on your weight loss plan and your way of life, you likely already have a night time regular that seems to be assisting, so the ones steps are the final matters to cowl earlier than entering into the miracle physical video games.

Step 1

Make nice your bed room is completely dark or as dark as feasible. A little moderate can alter your internal clock and the melatonin and serotonin levels produced for your pineal gland. Light tells your thoughts it is time to awaken, to get in movement. And however the truth that to you it can appear that a touch moderate can't interfere together with your sleep, believe me, it does. Tiny fragments of slight journey via your optical nerves and input at once for your hypothalamus.

Use blackout curtains, use a watch fixed masks, cowl your alarm clock, near your mattress room door, keep away from turning lights on at some stage inside the night time, even in case you go to the bathroom.

Step 2

Keep your room on the right temperature. This is amongst sixty five and 70 F tiers (18°C to 21°C). Too bloodless or too warmness equals awful sleep. When you sleep, your frame temperature decreases, such loads of scientists accept as true with that napping in a easy room might likely help sleep better because it imitates the decrease inside the frame's temperature.

Step three

Move the alarm clock faraway from your mattress, further to a few different electric powered powered gadgets. It's vital your clock is in a place wherein you may't see it; searching on the time nice reasons more stress, so skip it away. Electrical gadgets may have an effect at the pineal gland features and the producing of serotonin and melatonin. If it's possible, disconnect the circuit switch before you visit mattress.

Step 4

Reserve your bed exclusively for drowsing. If you're used to looking TV otherwise you figure for your bed, stop doing it. This can reason strain whilst you are trying to sleep; avoid doing the ones sports activities for your bed.

five Exercises For Better Sleep

The sporting sports activities you'll examine next may be used individually, or you can do them as a chain, it doesn't count as long as you do them correctly. It's viable you could fall asleep in the middle of one in all them, however good day, no hassle with that, proper?

#1 Short Workout

If you've got got hassle drowsing, this quick exercising can be very useful. You can comprise those physical sports to your middle of the night ritual and, in a short time, you'll see the distinction.

Exercise

1.Sit down within the ground and pass your legs. Breathe generally and regularly.

2.Now, vicinity your elbows on top of your knees and close to your eyes. Focus in for your breathing; sense how the air comes in through your nose, preserve it for two seconds and exhale slowly, very slowly thru your mouth. Don't pressure your respiration; permit it waft simply and slowly.

three.Still within the identical function, incline your trunk in advance fun your head. Breathe usually and frequently, in truth lighten up. Stay on this posture for a couple of minutes after which move again to the initial characteristic.

four.Extend your legs and try to touch the top of your toes collectively at the side of your palms. Relax your body, it doesn't depend in case you contact your feet or no longer, actually stretch your yet again and loosen up.

5.Now, sit down down on pinnacle of a pillow. Any pillow so long as you enjoy comfortable. Keep your again immediately. Use a tennis ball to massage the arch of your foot. Roll the ball from side to side below the arch of your foot.

#2 Relaxing Exercises

This is a contemporary relaxation workout, and the reality, it's excellent! You need to memorize the regular, and it may take a few days to do it, however after you examine it, you'll see how your frame softens and the anxiety for your muscular tissues disappears.

Another component you can do is document your self pronouncing this complete routine with a chilled and calming voice, and then you could be aware of it at night time time time.

Exercise

1.Lie all the manner down to your bed, discover a comfortable role and near your eyes.

2.Breathe generally; revel in your ft; middle your hobby on your ft. Be conscious of how plenty they weigh, lighten up your feet and revel in how they sink in your bed. Start together together with your toes after which float for your ankles.

3.Feel your knees; middle your interest on your knees. Be privy to techniques masses they weigh, lighten up your knees and experience how they sink on your bed.

4.Feel your legs and thighs; middle your interest in your legs and thighs. Be conscious of processes a extremely good deal they weigh, lighten up your legs and thighs and revel in how they sink on your bed.

5.Feel your stomach and your chest; center your interest for your stomach and your chest. Be privy to how a whole lot they weigh, loosen up your belly and your chest and experience how they sink in your bed.

6.Feel your buttocks; middle your attention for your buttocks. Be aware about strategies a whole lot it weighs, lighten up your buttocks and enjoy the way it sinks to your mattress.

7.Feel your fingers; center your interest in your hands. Be privy to methods masses they weigh, loosen up your palms and experience how they sink in your bed. Start with the thumb and maintain with the relaxation.

8.Feel your arms; middle your hobby to your arms. Be aware about how an awful lot they weigh, lighten up your palms and revel in how they sink on your mattress.

nine.Feel your shoulders; center your interest for your shoulders. Be aware of how a good buy they weigh, loosen up your shoulders and enjoy how they sink in your bed.

10. Feel your neck; middle your interest in your neck. Be privy to the manner a bargain it weighs, relax your neck and revel in the way it sinks for your bed.

eleven. Feel your head; middle your interest for your head. Be aware of its weight, lighten up your head and enjoy the way it sinks in your mattress.

12. Feel your mouth and your jaw; center your attention in your mouth and your jaw. Relax your mouth and pay precise interest in your jaw. Feel how your mouth and your jaw sink in your mattress.

thirteen. Feel your eyes; middle your interest to your eyes. Notice if there's anxiety to your eyes, consciously loosen up your eyes and enjoy how this tension movements faraway from your eyes.

14. Feel your cheeks; middle your attention in your cheeks. Notice if there's any anxiety for

your cheeks, consciously lighten up and flow into any anxiety away.

#three Breathing & Sleeping Exercises

Breathing is one of the abilities with greater have an effect on over your body; respiratory technique lifestyles! However, it is a few issue so herbal and automatic that we never reflect onconsideration on it as an answer. Breathing can be managed consciously, and via using doing it you could decrease strain and assist address insomnia and many one-of-a-type snoozing problems.

With primary breathing strategies, which encompass belly respiratory or diaphragmatic respiration, you could reduce muscular anxiety and do away with anxiety.

Exercise

1.For this workout, you may be mendacity all of the manner all the way down to your bed or but you feel comfortable.

2.Now, area one give up your stomach and the opportunity hand inside the top a part of your chest. This way you can revel in the diaphragmatic moves better.

3.Start thru breathing in deeply and slowly, believe the course the air makes internal your frame, try to visualize it. You will word how the air reaches your belly and how this "inflates." The thorax want to not glide. Contain the air inner for 3 seconds.

four.Relax any anxiety to your frame; reputation in your body. If your thoughts wanders to mind or troubles that's proper enough, clearly bring your hobby back to your body.

five.Exhale slowly on the identical time as you rely from 5 to 0, and focus on every bypass. Notice how each time you exhale air you enjoy increasingly more cushty.

6.Repeat this exercise five instances.

Important Note

It's vital to bear in mind to govern the velocity of your breathing as well as the quantity of air you inhale. Always examine a gradual and paused rhythm. If you inhale too quick or an excessive amount of air you could get dizzy. If this takes area, rest for a few seconds after which hold with the exercising.

#4 Getting Creative

If you are doing these sports activities as a series, you need to be feeling very cushty thru using now. But in case you're simply getting started out out out and there are some mind invading your mind then try this.

The idea of this workout is to popularity your interest on a tale or a picture on your thoughts so you can allow bypass of something that is demanding you.

Exercise

1.Visualize a scene or a tale, a few component you choose as extended as it's calming. For example, agree with a day on the seashore, a stroll in the park, or an area in which you experience snug; the concept is to discover some element to recognition your hobby on so that you permit circulate of your thoughts.

2.Be innovative, visualize each detail, attempt to experience the smells, see everything in your thoughts's eye, and permit bypass of your thoughts. If your thoughts drifts to an unpleasant or stressful perception, don't fight it, renowned it after which allow it move and keep doing your trouble.

3.I'll give you an example of the way it want to be, but once you get it, be creative and visit your chosen location inside the international, the one in in which you revel in maximum cushty.

four.Breathe in deeply and exhale slowly. Breathe interior and out, very slowly. Do this more instances.

5.Imagine you are in a big meadow; it's big and everything is green. You are mendacity down in the grass, and whilst you look up, you see a stunning, easy blue sky. The sky is terrific, there's no longer one cloud in it.

6.Feel the heady scent of a sunny day, sense the mild rays of the sun warming your face. Feel the air caressing your face, feel the sensation of a nice and brilliant day.

7.Breathe in deeply and exhale slowly, enjoy every second of this. Use all your senses to get inner this picture. It's absolutely you and the sky…

8.Stay interior your "mystery place" so long as you need to, overlook approximately the entirety else and enjoy this time with you.

#5 Silent Ears

This is an high-quality and effective workout; you can do it after your breathing exercising, after the innovative relaxation, or for my part.

Exercise

1.Place your arms inside the lower back of your head and loosen up. Breathe usually and regularly. Don't preserve your breath.

2.Now, together at the side of your thumbs near your ear canal. Do it through the usage of putting the thumbs in the ears.

three.Hear some detail? You might in all likelihood pay interest a rushing sound, if you do pay interest it this suggests you are doing it proper.

4.Stay in this feature for about fifteen mins, in fact listening to this sound.

5.Put your palms for your sides, breathe in deeply and exhale one time. Relax your arms and candy dreams!

Other Helpful Exercises

These following sports activities also can have a profound effect on assisting people get to bed.

Writing

Use a mag to write how your day have become, and try to be specific and write as many facts as you can take into account. You can also write the whole thing you propose on doing the following day, everything you need to do.

By doing this you loose your thoughts of pressure; you're telling your thoughts the whole lot is sorted. If you had a terrible day, with the resource of the use of writing down your emotions and the info you're dumping your mind out on paper. Everything is in that little magazine, no need to take it to mattress with you anymore.

Try to do that everywhere besides your mattress; inside the kitchen, for your desk, everywhere you want, honestly keep away from doing this in bed.

Checklist

If you are any such those who fear about things left to do, then this can be right for you. Make a brief listing of things you always worry about, like if the oven is turned off, the garage door closed, and matters left to do this might be annoying you when you are in mattress.

Sunglasses

A couple of hours earlier than your bedtime wear sunglasses. It could probable sound crazy to use shades round your home, however it sincerely works! By doing this, you trick your mind, and serotonin tiers will increase regularly and it'll be much less tough to fall asleep.

Bathroom Time

As I knowledgeable you earlier than, keep away from ingesting water a couple hours earlier than you visit bed. Hydrate your self within the course of the complete day, however no longer in advance than bedtime. Just in advance than stepping into mattress, visit the rest room, this reduces the possibilities of you waking up within the nighttime.

Socks?

Using socks at the same time as you sleep is truly as a whole lot as you. You realize your body, but some research indicates that folks who use socks throughout the night time sleep better. The cause for this? Well, your body temperature decreases at some diploma within the night time time time, and your feet are the part of the body with worst flow into and because of this they get bloodless. Keeping your toes heat will will permit you to sleep better

Stop it!

Stop operating at least more than one hours in advance than your bedtime; this will offer your mind time to loosen up earlier than getting into bed.

Relaxation

There are hundreds of interesting discs that assist you to sleep. You can pick out out a guided meditation, enjoyable music, or ocean sounds; something works for you.

Reading

If you take a look at a ebook, pick one this is soothing and no longer a mystery novel, as a manner to have the opposite impact.

Melatonin

You can boom your melatonin ranges truely, like by means of taking a solar tub at some point of the day. There also are a few melatonin supplements that permit you to.

Chapter 6: Power Nap

Nap: brief sleep or relaxation that ends in advance than getting into the deep sleep stages and is generally made after lunch or inside the middle of the day. There are many locations wherein the energy nap is a have to, like in Spain as an instance. The entire European u.S.A. Paralyzes from midday till four o'clock due to the reality everyone is in "siesta" (nap) time. Winston Churchill, Albert Einstein and John F. Kennedy had been huge fanatics of the energy nap.

These days a sleep is sort of a high priced; absolutely everyone desires to have time for a strength nap. But, there are various myths across the power nap, is it wholesome? Does it have an impact on sleep at night time time time? Let's get into this entire nap difficulty and solve the truth.

The Truth Behind The Power Nap

A power nap is an superb manner to live alert and lively. It allows recharge your highbrow batteries within the middle of the day, and enables growth popularity and creativity. There are many studies that endorse that a power nap can be beneficial, allow's take a look at them out.

Benefits of the Power Nap

•Improves cardiac functions and decreases high blood pressure

•Ability to enhance motor competencies

•Alleviates bodily anxiety

•Diminishes strain

•Improves studying and memory

•Increases creativity

•Augments productivity

•Improves temper

As you could see, a electricity nap may be beneficial on your health and your mind, however there are also some things you want to realise as a manner to revel in its benefits. Here are some tricks to nap the right way.

Keep it Short

When I say quick, I imply twenty-5 mins brief. According to research NASA published in 2011, a really best strength nap must be twenty-six mins. This have a look at changed into later confirmed with the useful resource of Harvard Medical School and the Mayo Clinic, who installation that a sleep need to last from twenty to thirty mins tops. If you sleep longer then you could wake up in the center of a deep sleep, and you may feel dizzy and could likely have problem dozing at night time time time.

Dark Room

To get the most out of your strength nap, try to do it in a dark room, or you can placed on an eye fixed masks.

Silence

Those naps in which you depart the TV on are not repairing at all. Voices on TV don't allow your mind to relaxation well, so if you could't get silence you higher consider skipping that nap.

Use Your Bed

I'm not announcing to jump into you PJ's or whatever, but the couch isn't an tremendous region to take a snooze. A top notch nap need to be mendacity down for your mattress.

Do it Early

If you want to sleep at night time time, you cannot nap at six o'clock within the midnight. The top notch time is amongst midday and 4 o'clock tops, if you nap for prolonged hours and do it too late you'll turn into a night time crawler.

Set Your Alarm

Turn your phone off so you revel in and make the maximum of your energy nap, but set your alarm, so that you don't exceed the twenty minute rule.

Again...Coffee

If you want to take a nap, don't drink coffee or it'll be not feasible to relaxation. If you could drink coffee, try to do it multiple hours in advance than taking your nap.

To Nap or Not to Nap?

A short nap within the direction of the day have that will help you recharge your power, but in instances in which you be bothered by way of insomnia or special napping issues naps are a no, no! If you be stricken by means of insomnia or different slumbering problems that maintain you from resting at night time, the incredible trouble is to visit mattress an hour early, and keep away from snoozing in any respect.

Chapter 7: Waking Up!

Now the whole thing about sleep, however we're now not completed but! Waking up in the right way is type of as crucial as sleeping nicely to start your day inside the first-class manner possible.

Besides one-of-a-type few sounds, the alarm clock is one of the maximum lousy sounds within the global! Humanity controlled to stay to tell the tale without those gadgets for loads of years, so why use them now? The answer is easy, right? Almost all people wishes an alarm clock to rouse every morning.

The truth is that when you have a healthful lifestyle, in case you recognize the desires and rhythms of your body, if you have an excellent enough night time recurring, and if you sleep properly, you don't need an alarm clock. Your body is perfectly able to waking up clearly every day on the identical time.

If you examine the education of this e book, in some time you may remove that traumatic alarm clock, but within the period in-between, there are a few options you need to awaken in a superb temper and glowing every day.

Alarm Clocks

The extraordinary manner to rise up is without loud alarms which could alter your nerves and purpose irritability at a few degree inside the day. Noisy alarms are unnatural, however can they've an effect in your fitness? The answer is positive. Loud alarms inside the morning can growth your blood stress and boom strain tiers.

Now, I need to speak a touch about the oh-so famous "snooze button." We have all been there, and the scene seems to replicate each day for lots; your alarm clock wakes you up and with horror you be aware it's time to wake up. You honestly need 5 extra minutes, so you push the magic button for you to will allow you to relaxation at least 5 more mins earlier than starting your day. Well...the usage of the snooze button regularly cannot be the extraordinary element to do; it is able to really initiate extra tiredness. What alarm clocks do is interrupt the herbal device of waking up. It's demanding sufficient, and in case you dispose of it with the snooze button, your napping cycle begins once more. So, the problem proper right right here is to attach and disconnect the mind time and again, this high-quality makes you extra tired.

Good Morning!

So, what's the high-quality manner to evoke inside the morning? There are many things you can do, allow's go through some of them.

Several studies have indicated that waking up with moderate may be beneficial for definitely all people, specifically to people who are practical to circadian rhythm modifications. Waking up with moderate is more healthful and extra herbal, gives you extra energy, and a higher temper for the duration of the day.

Light emits a message to the thoughts, so it regularly stops generating and liberating melatonin to your frame. This identical melatonin that we so desperately search for at night time is the equal we want to stop generating in large quantities all through the day to enjoy lively and unsleeping. With slight, the waking up method is gradual, more healthy, and this interprets into more energy and strength sooner or later of the day.

Nowadays, there are numerous alarm clocks which is probably capable of imitating the herbal dawn inner your room. These are very powerful; half an hour in advance than it gradual to upward push up the alarm clock begins offevolved illuminating your room grade by grade, until it reaches the brightness decided on.

You can also have an alarm clock that isn't always so noisy, if you are terrified of turning that off and falling returned asleep, you could set alarms, as an example one with a gentle enjoyable noise or music, and the second one as your returned up alarm.

After you open your eyes, the number one detail you have to do is wash your face with bloodless water, flip the lighting fixtures on so your mind starts releasing serotonin, pay interest to 3 upbeat tune and there you go, you are organized to have a remarkable day!

Chapter 8: What is Sleep and Why is it Important?

Most humans understand that sleep is crucial, however many do now not understand why. Sleep is a crucial a part of our each day routine, and it performs a crucial function in our trendy fitness and well-being.

Sleep is a herbal country of rest for our our bodies and minds. When we sleep, our our our bodies are capable of restore and regenerate cells, tissues, and organs. Sleep moreover lets in our brains to consolidate recollections and approach information. Most adults need among 7 and eight hours of sleep consistent with night time. However, a few human beings may also need extra or tons less relying on their age.

If you are no longer getting sufficient sleep, you can experience fatigue, irritability, temper swings, problem concentrating, and one-of-a-type physical and highbrow fitness issues. Lack of sleep can also reason weight gain, as it may increase your urge for food and decrease your metabolism.

Getting enough sleep is crucial to our trendy health and nicely-being. If you're not getting sufficient sleep, make certain to talk for your health practitioner to peer if there may be an underlying reason. There are also some clean way of life changes you can make to help beautify your sleep, collectively with preserving off caffeine before bed, putting in place a regular sleep time desk, and developing a soothing bedtime normal.

If you are not getting sufficient sleep, you may enjoy fatigue, irritability, mood swings, hassle concentrating, and different physical and highbrow fitness troubles. Lack of sleep also can bring about weight gain, as it may increase your appetite and reduce your metabolism.

If you're not getting enough sleep, ensure to speak to your doctor to look if there can be an underlying motive. There also are some easy lifestyle changes you could make to assist decorate your sleep, which consist of preserving off caffeine earlier than mattress, establishing a ordinary sleep time desk, and growing a chilled bedtime regular.

The Different Types of Sleep

There are extraordinary kinds of sleep: rapid eye motion (REM) sleep and non-speedy eye motion (NREM) sleep.

Rapid Eyes Movement (REM)

REM sleep is the section of sleep whilst you dream. Rapid Eye Movement, or REM, is a level of sleep characterised through the rapid motion of the eyes. This stage of sleep is crucial for every mental and bodily health.

During REM sleep, the mind is lively, and goals get up. The body is also paralyzed throughout this level, which prevents human beings from performing out their dreams. REM sleep is crucial for learning and memory. It additionally performs a function in regulating mood and energy ranges. Rapid eye motion sleep is commonly a lighter diploma of sleep than non-REM sleep. However, humans can no matter the truth that awaken from REM sleep if they will be disturbed.

REM sleep is essential for mind improvement and reminiscence. Most adults spend approximately 20% in their trendy sleep time in REM sleep.

REM Sleep Behavior Disorder

Rapid eye motion (REM) sleep conduct ailment is a situation that reasons human beings to behave inconsistently while they're asleep. People with this disorder also can shout, scream, or maybe lash out physical within the course of REM sleep, this is the inner most and maximum restful stage of sleep. REM sleep conduct sickness is idea to be because of a disconnection among the brain and the muscle mass in the path of REM sleep.

This can purpose humans performing out their desires, which may be volatile for every the man or woman and everyone else who is close by. REM sleep behavior disease (RBD) is a scenario that motives human beings to behave out their goals all through REM sleep. RBD is most in all likelihood due to a disruption inside the thoughts chemicals that control sleep and wakefulness. This can stand up because of neurologic issues, along with Parkinson's ailment or Lewy frame dementia. Other functionality motives encompass tremendous pills, genetic elements, and head accidents.

People with RBD often document brilliant and excessive desires, that would lead to them appearing out physical. This can variety from easy moves like kicking or punching to greater complex behaviors like the use of or cooking. In some instances, people with RBD had been regarded to injure themselves or others even as sleepwalking.

The accurate news is that REM sleep behavior sickness is treatable, and there are some of measures that may be taken to assist manipulate the situation. With proper remedy, human beings with this disorder can revel in an awesome night time time's sleep without fear of harming themselves or others.

Non-Rapid Eye Movement (NREM)

NREM sleep is a section of sleep characterised through sluggish and regular thoughts waves. It includes stages 1, 2, three, and four of sleep. NREM sleep is critical for bodily and highbrow recovery. NREM sleep has 4 extraordinary degrees, with every offering certainly one of a type thoughts wave styles.

•Stage 1 or N1

This degree is moderate sleep and lasts for approximately 5-10 minutes. Your eyes are closed during this degree, however if you were to be awoken, you'll likely experience as despite the fact that you had now not been asleep.

N1 is the lightest section of NREM sleep. You may additionally enjoy drowsy in some unspecified time in the future of this section, but you will be without trouble awoke. N1 sleep makes up approximately five-10% of your normal sleep time.

•Stage 2 or N2

The N2 diploma is also slight sleep, but it is a much deeper segment of NREM sleep. Your respiratory and coronary coronary heart charge slow down, and you are an lousy lot plenty less in all likelihood to be wakened within the path of this phase. N2 sleep makes up about 50-60% of your overall sleep time. Your eyes are regardless of the fact that closed throughout this phase. Brain waves at some point of this segment are called sleep spindles and K-complexes.

•Stage three or N3

N3 is a deeper NREM sleep stage, in which mind wave interest slows down even extra. It is tough to awaken from this degree of sleep. This is whilst your body maintenance and regenerates cells, tissues, and organs. N3 sleep is set 20-25% of your ordinary sleep time.

• Stage 4 or N4

Stage four: This is the internal most level of sleep, in which thoughts waves are very gradual. It is hard to evoke from this degree of sleep. Sleepwalking and night terrors frequently occur sooner or later of this degree.

It's vital to get all four degrees of NREM sleep, as every one performs a vital function on your frequent fitness and properly-being. When you do no longer get enough sleep, you can experience fatigue, irritability, temper swings, trouble concentrating, and other bodily and intellectual fitness issues. Lack of sleep can also cause weight benefit, as it may growth your urge for meals and decrease your metabolism.

If you aren't getting enough sleep, make sure to talk in your medical medical doctor to look if there may be an underlying cause. There also are a few easy life-style changes you could make to help enhance your sleep, which include fending off caffeine earlier than bed, organising a regular sleep schedule, and developing a calming bedtime habitual.

If you're a DIYer and you are struggling to get sufficient NREM sleep, there are some things you could do to help your self fall asleep and stay asleep. First, create a bedtime routine and maintain on with it as an entire lot as viable. This will sign on your body that it's time to wind down for the night time. Avoid caffeine and alcohol in advance than mattress, as those can intervene with sleep. Also, make certain that your bed room is dark, quiet, and funky – the ones are ideal situations for drowsing. Finally, in case you discover your self tossing and turning at night time time, escape from bed and do something calming until you sense sleepy all over again. Then, attempt going once more to mattress.

What are Circadian Rhythms?

Circadian rhythms are the every day fluctuations in our bodies that inform us whilst to sleep, awaken, and devour. They're controlled through the usage of manner of a "biological clock" inside the brain that continues track of the 24-hour day.

The critical cue for our herbal clock is light. When it's slight out of doors, our brains ship signs that make us experience large awake and alert. When it's darkish, our brains ship signals that make us sense sleepy. Our internal clocks also can be affected by different cues, like temperature and noise. But mild is the maximum crucial trouble in setting our circadian rhythms.

What takes location even as our circadian rhythms are out of sync?

If our circadian rhythms are out of sync, it may have an impact on our sleep, mood, and power stages. For instance, jet lag is a shape of circadian rhythm disease which could rise up while we journey to particular time zones.

Shift artwork is some other shape of circadian rhythm ailment that would arise at the same time as our artwork hours don't in shape up with our herbal frame clocks. This can result in fatigue, insomnia, and other health issues.

Getting enough mild within the path of the day and minimizing moderate publicity at night time time can help keep our circadian rhythms in sync. Taking everyday breaks, workout, and ingesting a wholesome weight loss program can also assist.

Factors Affecting Your Circadian Rhythm

There are many various factors that can have an impact for your circadian rhythm. Circadian rhythm is your frame's herbal way of regulating itself based totally on the time of day. It is managed with the aid of severa one in all a type hormones and enzymes and can be encouraged with the useful aid of a whole lot of outside factors. Light publicity, strain levels, excursion, and internal factors like age and scientific conditions can all play a characteristic in how nicely you sleep at night time time.

Some of the maximum commonplace outside elements that would have an effect on your circadian rhythm encompass mild publicity, stress stages, and excursion. Light publicity is possibly the maximum critical element, as it allows to modify the discharge of melatonin, it's one of the key hormones concerned in controlling your sleep cycle. Too an entire lot slight publicity can disrupt this device and result in insomnia or other sleep problems.

Stress stages also can have an effect on your circadian rhythm. When you are below strain, your frame releases a hormone known as cortisol, that could intervene with the ordinary functioning of your Circadian rhythm. This can motive issues like problem falling asleep or staying asleep, as well as feeling worn-out at some point of the day.

Travel can also disrupt your Circadian rhythm, especially if you're crossing time zones. This is due to the reality your frame's inner clock desires time to modify to the modern-day agenda. If you adventure regularly, you could locate it useful to paste to a ordinary sleep time table as a first-rate deal as feasible to reduce the disruption.

There are also some of inner elements which can have an effect for your circadian rhythm. These embody such things as your age, genetics, and clinical conditions. For instance, older adults typically have a tendency to have extra hassle napping at night time and can be much more likely to be by way of insomnia. And some clinical conditions, together with Parkinson's illness, can intervene on the facet of your frame's herbal sleep cycle.

If you're having trouble drowsing, it could be because of an underlying Circadian rhythm illness. There are some of high-quality treatment alternatives to be had, so it's far important to talk for your physician if you're experiencing persistent sleeplessness. With the proper treatment, you could help get your Circadian rhythm once more on route and experience a first rate night time time's rest. Circadian rhythm is an vital a part of your each day lifestyles. If you are having trouble napping, communicate to your physician about Circadian rhythm disorders and treatment options. With the right assist, you could get your Circadian rhythm once more on target and revel in an incredible night time time time's relaxation.

Maintaining a Healthy Circadian Rhythm

There are a few key topics you could do to make certain you keep a wholesome circadian rhythm.

First, get enough sleep. This might also moreover look like a no brainer, but getting sufficient brilliant sleep is critical for maintaining your circadian rhythm in check. Make positive to get as a minimum 7-8 hours of sleep every night time time, and if possible, hold on with a ordinary sleep time table.

Second, keep away from publicity to excellent slight at night. This manner restricting your display screen time in advance than mattress and making sure your mattress room is dark while you're attempting to find to sleep. Exposure to colourful mild can disrupt your frame's herbal sleep cycle.

Third, get some exposure to daytime for the duration of the day. This enables reset your internal clock and maintains your circadian rhythm on path. Try to get out of doors for a couple of minutes each day, even supposing it's truly to take a walk throughout the block.

By following the ones clean tips, you can assist make certain that your circadian rhythm stays wholesome and in balance.

The Importance of Sleep

Sleep is one of the most important elements of our lives. It lets in us recharge and prepares us for the next day. However, many humans do not get enough sleep, that may have a horrible effect on their health.

There is a lot of dialogue surrounding the importance of sleep. Some humans argue that getting enough sleep is crucial, even as others claim that you could get thru on much much less. However, the generation of sleep indicates that lack of sleep has a huge impact on our fitness. In this a part of this eBook, we are able to talk the dangers of no longer getting enough sleep and how it may affect your body and mind. We can also moreover even offer tips for enhancing your sleep hygiene and getting the most out of your shut eye!

There are some of fitness risks associated with not getting sufficient sleep. These encompass:

•Increased hazard of accidents and damage

•Impaired cognitive characteristic

•Decreased functionality to fight off contamination

•Weight advantage

•Depression

Not getting sufficient sleep may also have a brilliant effect in your physical and intellectual fitness. It is critical to ensure that you have grow to be enough relaxation every night time time time so you can function at your extremely good inside the course of the day! There are some subjects that you could do to decorate your sleep hygiene:

•Establish a ordinary sleep time desk through going to mattress and waking up at the same time every day. - Avoid caffeine, alcohol, and nicotine earlier than bedtime as they'll all intrude with sleep.

•Create a relaxing bedtime routine that will help you wind down in advance than sleep. This have to encompass analyzing, taking a tub, or listening to calming music.

•Make high quality that your bed room is darkish, quiet, and cool so that it is conducive to sleep.

If you're suffering to get sufficient relaxation, communicate to your clinical doctor about feasible answers. There are many stuff that can be completed to beautify your sleep conduct and ensure which you have become the first-rate near-eye which you need! Don't allow loss of sleep damage your health - make certain to get a few ZZZs this night time!

Sleep is essential for our not unusual fitness and properly-being, but so lots folks don't get sufficient of it. If you're not getting sufficient rest, it could have a excessive impact for your bodily and highbrow fitness. Be excellent to set up a regular sleep time desk, keep away from caffeine and alcohol earlier than bedtime, and create a relaxing bedtime routine. If you're although having trouble dozing, talk in your clinical health practitioner.

Eleven Reasons Why You Should Get Some Sleep!

The National Sleep Foundation reports that adults want amongst seven and 9 hours of sleep a day. Here are ten reasons why you need to make certain you get enough near-eye each night time.

•Sleep enables your coronary coronary heart. People who do now not get sufficient sleep are at risk for excessive blood stress and coronary coronary heart ailment. In the equal way that we emphasize the want to devour a low-fat meal for lowering ldl ldl cholesterol and retaining one's coronary coronary heart in remarkable form, wholesome snoozing behavior are also crucial to as a minimum one's nicely-being.

•Sleep allows your weight. Getting enough sleep facilitates modify the hormones that manipulate appetite, so you're an lousy lot less probably to overeat. According to numerous studies, getting a whole lot much less sleep than is usually recommended is associated with higher degrees of extra weight and an extended hazard of being overweight. It may additionally additionally additionally have an effect on how rapid you shed kilos at the same tIme as following a calorie-confined weight loss program.

•Sleep offers you electricity. When you're properly-rested, you've got extra power to get thru the day. According to sleep scientists, your body regenerates and restores itself commonly inside the route of the fourth sleep level, once in a while called slow-wave sleep or deep sleep. The propensity to supply ATP, our frame's electricity forex, is stepped forward in the direction of this era of sleep, which seems to be the sleep kingdom that improves strength the most.

•Sleep consolidates your memories. With the proper amount of sleep, your thoughts consolidates recollections from the day so that you can better recall them in some time. Recall and acquisition are each sports activities sports that show up while you are extensive awake. Regardless of the sort of reminiscence, sleep is notion to be critical for memory consolidation. The human mind appears to have a extra difficult time assimilating and remembering new understanding in case you do now not get enough sleep. Sleep contributes greater to intellectual readability than you can even understand.

•Sleep reduces pressure. When you are rested, you're higher capable of deal with pressure and anxiety. Indeed, getting enough sleep has been shown to significantly lessen tension signs and symptoms and symptoms and signs and symptoms and signs and symptoms thru improving your functionality to govern pressure and reply successfully. Particularly, getting a restful night time time of sleep may additionally additionally beautify your disposition, outlook, and mind-set.

•Sleep makes you more alert. A right night's sleep will help you be greater green and focused for the duration of the day. The accumulation of adenosine at the equal time as wakeful is thought to inspire the "choice to sleep." When we're clearly aware, adenosine builds up and remains immoderate. We seem greater wide awake on the identical time as we wake up due to the fact the body receives an possibility to take away adenosine from our machine on the equal time as we slumber.

•Sleep improves your pores and pores and skin. Getting sufficient sleep lets in your pores and skin live hydrated and reduces the appearance of wrinkles. While you sleep, your pores and skin produces new collagen, stopping sagging. According to dermatologists, snoozing is a massive a part of the pores and pores and skin mending device. The pores and pores and skin that has greater collagen is less attackable and much less at risk of wrinkles. Five hours a good deal less of sleep every night time time may additionally motive double as many wrinkles as seven hours.

•Sleep offers your thoughts a spoil. When you are asleep, your thoughts can relaxation and restore itself from the day's sports activities. Learning makes the thoughts's synaptic links stronger even as you're huge conscious, which will increase strength demands and inundates your brain with clean records. So that your mind can start over tomorrow, sleep allows your mind to refresh, assisting inside the integration of in recent times received information with entrenched memories.

•Sleep improves your mood. Getting enough sleep can assist decorate your temper and decrease pressure degrees. You're truly already aware of how sleep affects mood. You ought to revel in extra stressed out and grumpy tomorrow after a burdened night time time. When you have were given an splendid sleep, your temper normally regains its regular country. Research has established that even a chunk loss of sleep does have a massive effect on our moods.

•Sleep boosts your immune tool. Getting sufficient sleep can help enhance your immune device function and decrease your hazard of having ill. Our our bodies manufacture cytokines while we snooze, which might be immune reaction-targeted on proteins that assault infection and infection. T-cells, a kind of white blood mobile vital to the body's immunological response to infectious ailments, are also produced by means of the usage of the body when we sleep.

•Sleep allows you live targeted. If you are attempting to cognizance on a venture, getting sufficient sleep can assist improve your interest span and memory. Sleep permits in the development of a sharper thoughts. Considering how vital sleep is for memories and gaining knowledge of, this makes feel. Lack of sleep makes it tough to pay hobby and absorb smooth information. Additionally, the mind is not given enough time to save reminiscences for subsequent retrieval very well. So that you are prepared for what comes next, sleep permits your mind preserve tempo.

So there you have were given it! Ten reasons why you want to ensure you get enough sleep every night time time. By following these pointers, you could improve your trendy health and nicely-being.

How Much Sleep Do You Need?

How a first rate deal sleep do you want? It's a commonplace question and one that doesn't have a straightforward answer. Depending for your age, manner of lifestyles, and health, you can need anywhere from seven to nine hours of sleep every night time time.

There are many elements that would have an effect on how an entire lot sleep you need. Age is one of the maximum crucial factors. As we turn out to be antique, we usually require plenty a great deal less sleep. Lifestyle picks like working the night time shift or often travelling can also effect how an lousy lot sleep you need. And in the end, your famous health can play a feature in how hundreds near-eye you require.

If you're no longer getting enough sleep, there are a few matters you can do to try and beautify the scenario. First, test your lifestyle and word if there are any adjustments you could make to help you get greater rest. For example, in case you're on foot the night time time time shift, attempt to avoid caffeine after dinner and establish a everyday sleep schedule. If you regularly journey, try and ebook flights that arrive inside the morning so that you can adjust to the time alternate extra with out troubles.

And in the long run, if you're suffering with a health scenario that makes it difficult to sleep, communicate for your doctor about feasible remedies. They can be able to prescribe medicinal drug or recommend distinct strategies that will help you get the relaxation you want.

How to Prepare The Bedroom for a Good Night of Sleep

Investment in sleep will pay you in phrases of multiplied productivity, improved intellectual properly-being, and similarly strength in some unspecified time in the future of the day. But it's miles sometimes less difficult said than finished to attain a restful night time time's relaxation.

It is vital to exercise right "sleeping conduct" inside the moments preceding bedtime, which incorporates abstaining from exercising, alcohol, espresso, and precise stimulants.

However, even reputedly unimportant elements together with the lights in your home or the activities you engage in mattress at the same time as you're wide wide awake may have an effect in your capability to have a super middle of the night sleep. The splendid issue is that making the most of those elements can cause more rest and a honest extra exciting midnight habitual. Read immediately to learn the way they put together for mattress and advantage the splendid possible sleep.

1.Spend some time a laugh

You need to begin planning how and whilst you will unwind multiple hours preceding to retiring to mattress.

The majority of sleep specialists claim that maximum people are caught up on their art work after supper and they do not often time table their downtime earlier.

You do not generally require severa wind-down times. You are not required to drag to a halt notably a long manner earlier of the junction if the car is not shifting proper away. But on certain days, you're moving at 100 mph. You ought to offer your self sufficient time to tug to a halt.

Stress may be because of muddle. Making your bed each morning and putting dirty garments inside the cloth cupboard are subjects that, regular with research, may additionally help individuals get a higher night time time's sleep.

You need to pick out out your mattress companions carefully. Pets can intervene collectively collectively with your functionality to sleep and might boom your frame temperature if they share your mattress. Put animals far from the mattress if you could, and contemplate having them stay in a one-of-a-type room.

Setting up a relaxing nighttime ritual may additionally moreover beneficial resource in your intellectual healing after a disturbing day. After supper, take a walk to lighten up your head. If you discover that exercising lets you decompress, be careful to workout earlier than night time time so that the endorphins might not preserve you up later.

Self-care may additionally moreover include a spa go to in advance than going to bed. Apply night time time lotions with calming smells collectively with lavender, some element we have grown to relate with sleep, and feature a heat bath to easy off the dust and sweat you accumulated in some unspecified time within the future of the route of the day.

1.Reduce the depth of the thermostat and the lighting.

Scientists have determined that it takes the body approximately three hours to 4prepare for sleep. According to investigate, blue mild from gadgets like laptops, cell telephones, televisions, and LED lighting systems can intrude with the frame's ordinary manufacturing of melatonin. Unplug your gadgets on the final hour earlier than going to mattress, and think about moving your television and a few different gadgets to some other room.

By changing the temperature and lighting fixtures in your private home, you could train your device to get organized for sleep. The lighting fixtures must be steadily dimmed spherical the house starting at dinnertime, this is form of three hours before sleep for us. We are conscious that publicity to slight 2 to 3 hours preceding to night would probably reason your circadian rhythm, or internal clock, to enhance.

Melatonin, the biomolecular complex that indicators your body at the same time as it is sleep time, may be suppressed through using the presence of light.

A PS display's blue, cool light is particularly energizing as it has a tone that resembles sunshine. Downloading an software which include f.Lux, which modifies your show screen to generate hotter shades in the direction of midnight, is counseled if you have to carry out your PC at twilight.

Additionally, after supper, decrease the thermostat in your property through severa factors to cause a dip to your body temperature. The frame temperature is a physiological indication that aids inside the start of your sleep. If making a decision to take a bathtub in advance than bedtime, we advise doing so as a minimum sixty minutes earlier than really napping to offer your body time to wind down.

Decide on an appropriate temperature of your room. Most humans sleep maximum successfully in environments which might be amongst sixty-five and sixty-9 degrees due to the truth once they sleep, their frame temperature step by step decreases. Before retiring for the nighttime, if required, lower your thermostat.

Buy great window coverings. Black-out drapes and room-darkening coverings can block out mild from the out of doors worldwide and sell deeper sleep.

Keep a nightlight or flashlight handy if you ought to wake up at night time time time to prevent switching on lighting thinking about the reality that it may interfere along side your functionality to head decrease lower back asleep fast. By following those easy suggestions, you could prepare your mattress room for a high-quality night time's sleep. Sweet desires!

2.Keep Netflix away from your bed.

Your sleep want to function a snooze cause in addition to environmental indicators together with perfume, temperature, and moderate. You want to attempt to avoid sporting out non-sleep behaviors, which includes viewing

Netflix on your device, or in mattress, everyday with all 4 specialists.

The bed might not turn out to be the proper area for resting in case you are engaged in all of these specific sports activities in bed. It will become a place for the whole lot.

Can you dine in your restroom? We're asking the ones who've been taking into consideration, "Well, the mattress is comfier than the couch."

You also can moreover fall asleep greater speedy or even without the slump over your high-quality-cherished comedy show by using the use of the usage of teaching your mind that the bed is in which you sleep, without a doubt much like how the restroom is in which you've got interaction with exceptional herbal abilties.

To avoid going to bed in advance than it's far sleep time if you live in a tiny area, set apart a place for walking and any other for leisure. We endorse you to sit up atop the covers or possibly rotate your frame to physical make a distinction in your sleep posture if you cannot keep away from spending some aware time sleeping in bed. three.Leave your bed in case you're demanding your self wide unsleeping.

If you can not get to sleep, staying aware at night time time will clearly cause greater careworn nights in the future. If you have got been unable to nod off for over twenty to thirty mins after retiring to bed, upward push up.

Leave your mattress as quickly as you revel in wakened; many patients are attempting to find recommendation from this sense due to the truth the "second wind." The mind will in the long run nod off in case you press it too tough. So pass, input another room until you nod off once more, then skip lower back in your bed. And then repeat it as regularly as crucial.

Numerous human beings claim that they experience practising yoga or meditation at the floor beside their beds till when they experience drowsy another time. Keep a pocket ebook nearby your bedside so you may also moreover take notes of any particular troubles or assets you want to get finished. Instead of using her cellular phone or pc to file them, write them on a bit of paper to reduce the hazard of being sidetracked.

You may also furthermore prevent yourself from getting lured into social media at some point of a pressured night time time by way of setting your mobile phone in flight mode. We endorse getting one hour of a cellular phone-unfastened period in advance than going to mattress to save you you from viewing whatever that would motive you to live concerned.

Sleep first-class can be significantly progressed by means of making little adjustments. Most people realize that they want to try to get great sleep, however few understand the manner to prepare their bedrooms for sleep nicely.

The first step is to create a nap-quality environment to your mattress room. This method keeping the room darkish, quiet, and funky. You may additionally moreover furthermore need to go through in thoughts the use of a white noise machine or earplugs to block out any out of doors noise.

Next, you may need to make certain your mattress is cushty and alluring. This approach having easy sheets which can be freed from any wrinkles or lumps. You also can additionally want to characteristic a further blanket or pillow for delivered consolation.

Finally, you may need to create a pre-sleep habitual to help you relax and wind down for the night time. This should probably encompass analyzing a ebook, taking a tub, or writing in a magazine.

Right under, we're going to offer you with some recommendations on a manner to create a nap-pleasant surroundings and make sure your mattress is snug so you can get the amazing sleep possible.

Why You Should Switch off the Lights Before Sleeping

There are loads of unique reasons to update the lighting fixtures off earlier than snoozing. For one, it is wholesome for you. Exposure to slight suppresses the manufacturing of melatonin, a hormone that lets in alter sleep. It's great to preserve your publicity to moderate at a minimal in case you're looking to get an high-quality night time's relaxation.

Also, it is in truth more enjoyable to sleep in darkness. This permit you to doze off faster and stay asleep longer. It is excellent to exchange the lighting off earlier than mattress in case you're searching for to get the most out of your sleep. That stated, let us take a look at out ten sturdy reasons why it's far essential to replace off the lighting in advance than sleeping:

Four Reasons Why You Should Switch Off the Lights Before Sleeping

1.Healthy sleep: Switching the lights off earlier than you sleep will assist you to get a more fit night time time's sleep. Studies have tested that publicity to slight can disrupt your body's natural sleep-wake cycle, making it more difficult to go to sleep and stay asleep. As such, you want to make certain the lighting fixtures are off so you will have the extremely good night time's rest.

2.Lights off: Studies have proven that an excessive amount of slight publicity can negatively impact your mood and strength levels. Turn the lights off earlier than bedsit indicators for your frame that it's time to wind down and put together for sleep if you're seeking to keep away from feeling groggy and gradual in the morning. This will assist you to go to sleep more rapid and enjoy a deeper, more restful sleep.

3.Save coins: Keeping the lighting off at night time time can also assist you save to your strength bill. If you're searching out strategies to reduce costs, that could be a easy but effective way. This technique that you could appreciably reduce your electricity payments if you prevent the vain usage of devices and lights at the same time as they may be now not wanted.

4.Reduce strain: Getting an first rate night time's sleep can help lessen stress and promote higher regular fitness. If you are struggling with stress, switching off the lights in advance than mattress can be useful. This element is mainly greater mentioned in human beings which is probably very touchy to mild. The truth is that the absence of lights allows sleep for almost every body in the global.

Are You Feeling Tired After a Midnight Awakening?

It may be virtually annoying to evoke in the dead of night, mainly if it takes vicinity regularly. For REM sleep cycles, it is essential to have a whole night time's rest. The frame dreams a while to transition once more into speedy eye movement sleep after a sleep disturbance, which could possibly depart you feeling sleepy the following day.

What Prompts Midnight Awakening?

You may be woken up inside the middle of the night for a number of causes. Some can be dealt with easily at domestic. You can also preference to visit your health practitioner for others.

Sleep Apnea

You can frequently wake up up at some point of the night time time or revel in hassle respiration in case you've got sleep apnea. Most patients of sleep apnea are ignorant of the disruptions to their sleep.

Even if you're no longer aware about it, you may enjoy sleepy at a few stage inside the day. Other big signs of sleep apnea include:

• respiratory closely in the course of sound asleep

• loud night breathing

- Daytime hobby issues

- Morning migraines

Your scientific physician will probably propose that you visit a snooze sanatorium to accumulate a assessment. You is probably located on the facility whilst you sleep. Additionally, a few physicians recommend home sleep finding out.

Sleep Apnea Therapies

• Airway strain contraptions: These devices are applied at the same time as you sleep. The device uses a sleep masks to inject a small quantity of oxygen into the lungs. A very popular device used to cope with that is the CPAP (non-stop effective airway stress). Alternatively, you can want to utilize distinctive gadgets together with bilevel immoderate first-rate strength airway strain and Auto-CPAP.

• Oral devices. Your dentist commonly has get proper of access to to those devices. The oral devices, which feature by using way of the use of lightly pushing the jaw beforehand and developing the airway within the course of sleep, are similar to mouthguards.

• Surgery. Surgery as a way for curing sleep apnea is usually the ultimate inn for sleep specialists. The sorts of strategies involve tissue excision, jaw realignment, implants, and nerve stimulation.

Night terrors

Even despite the fact that human beings experiencing sleep terrors seldom awaken, they will supply the impact of being conscious. Night terror patients often act out their fears aloud in their sleep, thrashing and screaming. There is a stunning emergence of focus, and the slumbering person may additionally moreover moreover even upward thrust up from mattress all of a surprising.

Those experiencing sleep terrors commonly don't undergo in thoughts what transpired till they wakeful day after today Sleep terrors afflict greater or plenty less 40 percent of children and a lower huge style of adults.

Children frequently triumph over this case with the useful resource of themselves. Nevertheless, you have to alert your physician in case you be conscious that your teen's sleep terror is worsening each day. Speak together collectively with your scientific health practitioner if:

• Events pose a danger to the sleeper

• Your infant studies episodes extra often

• your kid suffers terrors that frequently disturb them

• recurrent incidents persist after children

• The teenager sleeps excessively inside the path of the day.

Chapter 9: What is Sleep Routine and Why is it Important?

A sleep habitual is a difficult and fast of conduct which you perform every night before going to mattress. The motive of a snooze regular is to assist prepare your body and thoughts for sleep and to create an surroundings that is conducive to restful sleep. Sleep carrying events can variety from man or woman to character. Still, there are some not unusual factors that are frequently blanketed, along facet winding down for half-hour earlier than bed, disconnecting from electronics indicates, reading, or taking a bath.

There is not any character-length-fits-all technique to growing a snooze habitual, however there are some preferred pointers that may be found so that it will create a wholesome ordinary. First, it's miles critical to installation regularity and maintain on with a regular time desk. This way going to mattress and waking up at the same time each day, even on weekends. It also can be useful to create a pre-sleep ritual that signs in your frame that it's time to wind down and put together for sleep.

This need to comprise dimming the lighting fixtures, turning off digital suggests, and reading or taking a tub. By following the easy guidelines we'll communicate under, you may create a wholesome sleep everyday that will help you get the restful sleep you need.

Reasons Why You Should Have a Healthy Sleep Routine

Having a wholesome sleep ordinary is important to your normal health and nicely-being. When you get sufficient extraordinary sleep, it could help enhance your temper, beautify your energy degrees, and promote better bodily health. Sleep is also vital for intellectual health, supporting to reduce pressure and tension degrees.

There are a few key matters you could do to set up a healthy sleep recurring. First, try to visit bed and wake up on the equal time each day. This will assist modify your frame's natural sleep cycle. Secondly, create a calming surroundings in your mattress room that promotes appropriate sleep hygiene. This method ensuring the room is dark, quiet, and funky - all elements that can help you go to sleep greater without issues. And ultimately, keep away from the use of digital gadgets inside the bedroom, because the blue light emitted from video display units can disrupt your sleep.

So why is having a wholesome sleep ordinary essential in your health? Getting enough pleasant sleep is crucial for principal a glad and healthy life. By following those easy guidelines, you may decorate your acquainted health and properly-being - each physical and mentally.

Why You Should Have a Great Sleep Schedule

A ordinary sleep agenda is important on your ordinary fitness. When you hold on with a ordinary sleep time table, you deliver your body the threat to repair itself and recover from the day's sports activities. This can help improve your temper, growth your strength tiers, and reduce stress.

If you've got were given were given a normal sleep agenda, you're additionally much more likely to get enough deep sleep. Deep sleep is even as your frame does maximum of its restore paintings, so it's crucial in your bodily health. Getting enough deep sleep can assist enhance your immune device, coronary heart fitness, and cognitive characteristic.

It can be difficult to paste to a regular sleep time table, specially if you have a hectic manner of existence. But there are some matters you could do to help yourself out. Make high-quality to wind down for at the least an hour in advance than mattress, and avoid using displays (consisting of your cell smartphone) in the hours main as a lot as sleep. Establish a calming bedtime normal, and stay with it as plenty as feasible. And ultimately, try to create a sleep-best environment in your bed room – darkish, cool, and quiet.

If you can determine to a ordinary sleep time table, you'll be doing all of your health a need. So deliver it a attempt this night and be aware how you sense!

How to check and Find a Good House Routine

Are you having trouble sleeping at night time? You're not on my own. Many humans warfare to get sufficient restful sleep on a regular basis. There are pretty lots of of factors you can do to help discover the right sleep habitual for you.

First, bear in mind your sleep conduct and the manner they'll be impacting your sleep great. Are you staying up too late at night time or spending an excessive amount of time looking at video show devices before mattress? These habits should make it more difficult to doze off and live asleep all through the night time time time.

Second, take a look at your bed room environment. Is it dark, quiet, and cool? These are first-class conditions for drowsing, so try to create an environment that promotes rest.

Third, set up a ordinary sleep time table thru going to bed and waking up on the identical time every day. This will assist alter your frame's natural sleep rhythm and make it less hard to doze off and live asleep.

Finally, attempt some rest strategies before bedtime that will help you wind down and put together for sleep. This may also need to encompass reading, taking a tub, or operating towards deep respiratory bodily sports. By following those pointers, you may assist find out the right sleep habitual for you and get the restful sleep you need.

There are a number of specific sleep physical sports obtainable, and it can be tough to understand which one is proper for you. But following a sleep recurring is critical for getting the maximum restful sleep possible. Here are a few hints on the way to find and look at a nap habitual it's miles proper for you:

1.Figure out how loads sleep you want. Everyone's sleep needs are one in all a type, so it's far critical to decide out how a tremendous deal sleep you in my view want as a way to sense properly-rested. You can do that with the useful resource of preserving song of what number of hours of sleep you get every night time for every week or and then averaging out the quantity of time you sleep. This will give you a awesome idea of the manner a good buy sleep you need on a nightly basis.

2.Find a nap recurring that works for you. Once you apprehend how a first-rate deal sleep you want, you can start seeking out a snooze ordinary that will help you get that quantity of sleep. There are loads of one in every of a type carrying events to be had, so it is crucial to locate one which suits your lifestyle and time table. If you have got were given got hassle slumbering at night time, as an instance, you may possibly need to strive following a bedtime routine that includes winding down for 1/2 of-hour earlier than going to mattress.

three.Stick for your sleep everyday. Once you have got located a snooze everyday that works for you, it is important to paste to it as an awful lot as viable. This method going to bed and getting up at the equal time every day, even on weekends and vacations. It additionally may be beneficial to avoid naps sooner or later of the day, as they will make it more difficult to sleep at night time time.

Following a snooze, regular is critical for buying the maximum restful sleep viable. There are hundreds of brilliant workout routines out there, so it's far vital to discover one which fits your manner of lifestyles and time table. Once you've got placed a ordinary that works for you, stick to it as a fantastic deal as possible for the exceptional outcomes.

20 Tips for Best Sleep Routine

1.Keep a ordinary sleep time desk: Go to mattress and awaken at the same time every day, even on weekends. This will help alter your frame's natural sleep rhythm. As you have already study, a healthy character calls for not less than seven hours of middle of the night sleep each night time. Most people can nod off for a chunk upwards of 8 hours and yet sense refreshed. On weekends, go to your bed and upward push at the identical hour every day. Consistency strengthens the sleep-wake pattern for your body.

2.Create a pre-sleep ordinary: Do the same topics each night time time in advance than bed to signal for your frame that it's time to wind down. For example, take a warm temperature bath, look at a e-book, or be privy to calming music. Setting up and sticking to a normal nighttime normal will assist you in getting the sleep you require to rouse feeling snug and wide wide unsleeping. Despite the truth that it sounds hard to take a look at this recommendation, working closer to proper sleep hygiene will help you set up a nightly ordinary and boom a higher sleep cycle.

3.Avoid caffeine and alcohol in advance than mattress: Both of these materials can disrupt sleep. Caffeine must be prevented for at least six hours earlier than bedtime, even as alcohol need to be confined to 1 drink in line with day. Experts endorse that we should keep away from taking alcohol or caffeine 3 hours earlier than drowsing. They opine that on the equal time as alcohol can be first of all sedating in order that we doze off brief as soon as we take it may interfere with our regular sleep cycle. Caffeine, on the other hand, has the alternative impact. It can hold us aware longer than traditional. Since every substances tamper with our herbal sleep cycles, it's miles incredible to avoid them usually.

4.Create a snug sleeping surroundings: Make powerful your mattress room is darkish, quiet, and funky. A comfortable mattress and pillow also can assist sell restful sleep. The first step in getting your frame to loosen up is to make certain your sleep surroundings is clean and free of any interruptions. A treadmill, busy painting, or critical process office work are only some times of uncomfortable reminders of your responsibilities that would hold you up at night time time. Alternatively, make an effort to maintain your area litter-free and minimally decorated.

five.Get regular exercise: Exercise can beautify sleep outstanding through helping to modify the body's herbal sleep rhythms. However, it's superb to keep away from strenuous exercise close to bedtime as this could interfere with sleep. According to trendy day research, exercising allows people with insomnia and sleep issues. Aerobic workout appears to have a similar effect on sleep as sleeping medicinal pills.

6.Limit show display time earlier than bed: The blue mild emitted thru monitors can disrupt the body's natural sleep hormones. It's fine to avoid display time for as a minimum an hour earlier than bedtime. Using devices at the same time as seeking to sleep may also shorten your sleep and make it more difficult to nod off. There are diverse reasons for this: You can also experience inspired if you use a show thirty minutes earlier than dozing. As noted in advance, blue mild from televisions, computer systems, drugs, and phones can also inhibit melatonin manufacturing and eliminate tiredness.

7.Relax in advance than mattress: Stress and tension may want to make it difficult to doze off and live asleep. Try relaxation strategies along side deep respiratory or present day muscle relaxation that will help you float off to sleep. A lot of parents have a chilled addiction earlier than mattress. Another commonplace approach for treating insomnia is to exercising rest techniques earlier than bed, that have been established to enhance the great of your sleep.

8.Avoid naps during the day: Napping can intrude with middle of the night sleep. If you need to nap, limit it to half-hour or less and reap this early inside the day. Most humans's exceptional of nocturnal sleep is generally unaffected via short naps. However, taking a sleep could make your awful nice of sleep or insomnia at midnight worse. Nocturnal sleep ought to properly be hampered via prolonged or ordinary naps.

9.Eat a healthy weight loss program: Eating a balanced food regimen can help promote restful sleep. Avoid consuming large food in advance than bedtime, as this may cause indigestion and disrupt sleep. Your vitamins and weight-reduction plan may have an effect on the fitness of your night time's sleep, and a few elements and beverages also can make it more or a extraordinary deal lots less tough if you need to achieve the rest you deserve. Getting suitable enough sleep is likewise related to keeping a wholesome frame weight, that is high-quality for the ones trying to reduce weight.

10. Keep a snooze diary: Tracking your sleep behavior permit you to understand ability troubles and make vital adjustments to decorate your sleep pleasant. The diary permits for the calculation of overall hours of sleep through monitoring sleep. Individuals

can hit upon sleep disturbances and one-of-a-kind factors that would have an effect at the wonderful in their sleep through keeping a snooze magazine. Finding specifics about practices that intrude with sleep might show patterns that beneficial resource within the rationalization of napping issues.

11. Limit exposure to moderate at night time: Exposure to mild can disrupt the body's herbal manufacturing of melatonin, a hormone that lets in adjust sleep. To sell restful sleep, keep away from first-rate lights in the night and keep your bed room dark. The absence of moderate is critical for falling asleep and staying asleep. The frame gets a key sign that it is essential to shut eye while there is no slight. The herbal device that controls sleep-wake durations, called the frame's herbal "sleep clock," is altered on the equal time as the frame is exposed to mild at inappropriate durations. This interference influences every the satisfactory and quantity of sleep.

12. Use cushty sheets: A nicely night time's sleep is based upon at the pleasant of the mattress sheets. Your bed's consolation would possibly depend heaps at the nation of your covers. Sheets which are too heat or too bloodless can disrupt sleep. Use sheets made from herbal fibers which includes cotton or linen that will help you stay cushty at some stage in the night. Our our bodies produce heat at night time, so it's miles essential to select apparel that does not maintain it. The ability of mattress sheets to resource in tension and strain bargain is a few different high-quality advantage. Several humans discover that honestly lying on a cushty mattress makes them snug, and this may assist reduce fashionable physical stress.

13. Get up and bypass spherical each few hours: Sitting or lying in a unmarried role for too prolonged can result in stiffness and soreness. To lessen the chance of pain, stand up and circulate spherical each few hours. When you do this, it is able to continually translate to better sleep thinking about you

can't be experiencing the pain that consists of having body pains even as sleeping.

14. Take breaks within the course of extended intervals of sitting: If you have to take a seat down for lengthy durations of time, take common breaks to upward thrust up and stretch your frame. This will assist beautify flow into and decrease the hazard of ache. When you try this, it could usually translate to higher sleep on the grounds that you may not be experiencing the discomfort that is composed of getting body pains on the same time as snoozing.

15. Adjust your napping function: Your slumbering posture has a large impact at the first-rate of your sleep; therefore, in all likelihood it's time to change. Different napping postures offer severa advantages. You can also additionally want to trade positions to govern any ache further to one of a kind medical troubles you're coping with. Sleeping to your decrease again permits your head, neck, and resolution to rest in a

impartial function. This can help lessen the chance of pain and sell restful sleep. 16. Use a pillow that permits your head and neck: A pillow this is too excessive or too low can reason neck ache. Choose a pillow that helps your head and neck in a snug characteristic. One of the incredible options inside the market is a cervical pillow. The truth that cervical pillows absolutely enhance sleep with better posture is a large gain. By soothing and stabilizing stiff shoulder and neck muscle organizations and boosting blood circulate on your skull, similarly they ought that will help you sleep higher.

17. Stretch or do relaxation bodily sports in advance than mattress: Stretching or doing relaxation wearing activities together with yoga can help sell sleep with the aid of decreasing muscle tension and stress. Falling asleep more rapidly after a few moderate stretching can help when you have problem sleeping off. Before going to mattress, do some slight stretching to enhance your fashionable fitness and sleep duration. Prior

to going to bed, keep away from excessive or prolonged stretching because of the fact this can disrupt your sleep. Additionally, it can boom blood go with the flow and lessen muscular stiffness, which both helps restful sleep and muscular repair. The more you are able to permit your system to unwind in advance than bed, the higher you can sleep.

18. Avoid strolling in bed: Working in bed can create an association between the bed room and wakefulness, making it more tough to fall asleep. If possible, create a committed workspace in every different room to help you wind down in advance than bed. Medical professionals concur that running on some element on the same time as on your bed also can intrude along with your sleep cycle and probably reduce your productiveness. Not to feature that it would damage your dozing feature, leaving you with ugly aches and pains that a excellent workplace setting may additionally need to have avoided.

19. Reserve the mattress for sleep and sex: The mattress room have to be a place for rest and sleep. Avoid the use of the bed for sports at the side of searching tv or operating on the laptop. Lots of sleep professionals count on that jogging on a few issue while to your bed might also moreover moreover intervene along aspect your sleep cycle and potentially lessen your productivity. Not to add that it might wreck your sound asleep posture, leaving you with unpleasant aches and pains that a excellent place of business putting have to have averted. To this end, it's far vital to order your bed for sex and sleep and not to apply it as your workspace.

20. Follow a ordinary sleep time desk: Going to mattress and waking up on the same time each day can help adjust the body's herbal sleep rhythm. Try to stick to a ordinary sleep agenda, even on weekends and vacations. Maintaining a everyday sleep schedule, particularly within the route of your weekends, maintains the body's herbal clock on the right song and might make it a great

deal much less difficult as a way to evoke and nod off. Even even though putting in the suitable sleep time desk is tough due to each day duties, even modest changes must have a big effect on how nicely you sleep.

Chapter 10: Best Food to Eat Before and After Sleeping

Sleep and nutrients are important factors of our lives. Sleep is critical for our bodily and emotional fitness, on the same time as unique nutrients is top to keeping a healthful frame weight and stopping persistent ailments. In this chapter, we're capable of find out the connection among sleep and nutrients. How does sleep have an effect on our nutritional consumption? And how does what we devour assist us get an splendid night time time's sleep?

When we are sleep deprived, our our our our bodies crave energy-dense, high-carbohydrate components. This is due to the truth whilst we are worn-out, our our bodies launch the hormone ghrelin in response to low blood sugar stages—ghrelin signs to our brains that we are hungry and want to eat. As a result, we may discover ourselves achieving for sugary snacks or comfort meals whilst we revel in exhausted. Sleep deprivation also can bring about cravings for salty and fatty ingredients.

While those sorts of meals may additionally deliver us a transient power improve, they'll be not high-quality for our fundamental health. In truth, research have proven that individuals who devour a healthy eating plan excessive in sensitive carbohydrates and saturated fats are much more likely to enjoy terrible sleep. This is due to the fact the ones food can cause spikes in blood sugar levels, that could cause stressed nights.

So, if you're seeking to decorate your sleep, it is essential to focus on ingesting a nutritious weight loss plan. Complex carbohydrates, together with whole grains, beans, and veggies, are a notable supply of slow-release electricity that could assist hold blood sugar tiers robust in the direction of the night time time. And protein-rich food like lean meats, nuts, and seeds include amino acids that promote relaxation and help us sleep extra soundly.

Of path, all people's our bodies are one-of-a-kind, and there's no person-length-suits-all approach to nutrients. But by paying attention to how your eating regimen influences your sleep patterns, you can make certain you have become the vitamins you want to help a brilliant night time time's rest.

20 Foods to Can Help You Sleep Well

There are pretty a few blessings to ingesting the right meals before sound asleep. Sleep is crucial for our normal health, and eating the right substances can assist us get a higher night time's sleep. Here are 20 food to consume earlier than drowsing.

Eating a slight night time time dinner is regularly advocated for people who've hassle napping. Some studies indicates that eating too close to bedtime can intervene with sleep. One look at found that individuals who ate their nighttime meal plenty a good deal less than hours in advance than bedtime took longer to nod off and had more trouble staying asleep in the path of the night time in comparison to people who ate their midnight meal three or extra hours in advance than bedtime.

If you're searching out a slight night time dinner opportunity, try a few soup or a salad. Both options are easy on the stomach and acquired't leave you feeling too complete before bed.

Another meals with the intention to can help you sleep better is cherries. Cherries are a herbal supply of melatonin, that's a hormone that permits adjust sleep. A small have a test placed that individuals who drank cherry juice two times a day for 2 weeks slept an average of 34 minutes longer every night time time in comparison to those who didn't drink cherry juice.

If you're not eager on cherries, special substances contain melatonin as nicely, which includes bananas, tomatoes, walnuts, and oats. Try this kind of alternatives if you're seeking out a snack earlier than mattress to help you sleep.

Some studies indicates that first-rate factors can help lessen the hazard of nightmares. One observe decided that those who ate a high-protein meal earlier than bed were an awful lot a lot much less probable to have nightmares in evaluation to folks who ate a carbohydrate-rich meal.

So if you're searching out a bedtime snack to help you sleep and reduce the threat of nightmares, attempt some protein-rich options like nuts, seeds, tofu, or tempeh.

If you're someone who frequently wakes up in the middle of the night feeling thirsty, you could need to attempt eating a few chamomile tea in advance than mattress. Chamomile is a herb that has lengthy been used as a herbal remedy for insomnia and anxiety. One check observed that those who drank chamomile tea for two weeks slept a median of 32 minutes longer each night time time time in assessment to those who didn't drink chamomile tea.

There are many different food that can help you sleep higher, together with almonds, kiwi, honey, and lavender. So in case you're searching out a manner to get a better night time's sleep, strive incorporating a number of those substances into your diet. Sleep is crucial for our normal health, and ingesting the proper food can assist us get the relaxation we want. Try the ones 20 components earlier than slumbering and notice how they arrive up with the outcomes you want.

Some humans find out that their sleep improves once they keep away from caffeine in the evenings. If you're looking for a bedtime drink that will help you sleep, try herbal tea or decaffeinated espresso.

If you're having problem snoozing, there are numerous matters you can try to help beautify your sleep. Creating a bedtime habitual and heading off caffeine in the nighttime can help. And if you're looking for a snack earlier than mattress that will help you sleep, do that kind of 20 options. Sleep is vital for our common fitness, so it is without a doubt surely well worth taking the time to discover what works for you. Try those elements in advance than dozing and notice how they help you get a higher night time time's rest.

1.Milk

It works, this is why eating a heat glass of milk previous to bedtime is a popular. The hormone that promotes sleep, melatonin, is really present in cow's milk. Milk from cows which can be milked at some stage in the nighttime has greater melatonin, that is transferred to us whilst we drink milk in advance than sound asleep.

A cup of malt-enriched milk can artwork as properly if a desired glass of milk could not precisely do the magic. This kind o milk is prepared from a powdered mixture of sugar, malted barley, malted wheat, and wheat flour. Malted milk is stated to help with sleep as it incorporates vitamins B and D. According to at least one research, ingesting malted milk earlier than night time minimizes sleep disruptions.

Prepare It Before Bedtime: Before going to mattress, drink a few undeniable or malt-enriched milk. Or, have a few milk and cereal.

2.Kiwi

In area of extra famous culmination, the kiwi fruit is every so often omitted. This tiny fruit is a effective supply of nutrients and minerals that sell sleep. In a positive research, members located that ingesting kiwis one hour before bedtime ended in an additional sleep hour. Kiwis are wealthy in serotonin and weight loss plan C, every of which is probably sleep-inducing substances. Eat one kiwi before bedtime, each through the use of itself, with strawberries, or some one of a kind tropical quit end result.

three.Nuts

Pistachios, walnuts, and almonds are some examples of tree nuts which might be superb snacks. These crispy snacks are awesome for selling sleep. Magnesium, melatonin, and zinc—all substances discovered in nuts—can useful aid with sleep. According to as a minimum one studies, older men and women with insomnia benefited from taking nutritional supplements containing the same factors that nuts do to sell sleep.

Eat one handful of your selected tree nut in advance than bedtime, or devour a few mixed nuts or path combo as a snack.

four.Fatty Fish

Fish has lengthy been hailed for its wonderful effects on health. Fatty fish is an important a part of a coronary heart-healthy diet for the reason that it's miles excessive in weight-reduction plan D and protein. A tin of sardines or one salmon on occasion can also play a essential function at some point of napping.

According to one research, people who ate up salmon 3 instances consistent with week slept appreciably higher than those who didn't.

Additionally, the researchers found that fatty fish has extensive portions of omega-three fatty acids and vitamins D, which assist serotonin production.

For supper, grill a few salmon or different fatty fish, then for a nighttime snack, munch on a tuna can.

five.Rice

Rice is a number of the most famous food ate up global, and it will surely beneficial useful resource on your potential to get some sleep. Rice is one instance of a carbohydrate-wealthy meal this is wealthy in sugar and is frequently debatable in terms of nutrients. While consuming excessive rice might probable harm your waistline, studies advise that it can additionally decorate your sleep. Other carbohydrates with a big glycemic index, or individuals who brief spike blood sugar, are related to lots an awful lot much less restful sleep.

According to to a have a look at on Japanese adults, people who eat rice regularly sleep lots higher than individuals who devour more noodles and bread. Eat rice in advance than drowsing. For your dinner, prepare some stir-fries, and for dessert or a light snack, eat rice pudding.

6.Tart Cherries

Tart cherries, candy maraschino's bitter cousin, offer a number of medically mounted advantages, which encompass supporting with joint pain remedy and sleep. Whole tart cherries, nutritional supplements, and juice are all available available on the market. Tart cherries have antioxidant houses that resource in sleep marketing and immoderate melatonin levels that promote the protection of circadian rhythms.

In a 2018 studies on some of human beings, it have turn out to be proven that the respondents who took glasses of this fruit juice every day slept longer and further correctly than the individuals who didn't.

Drink one glass of clean tart cherry juice for some hours earlier than going to mattress. The juice's very sour taste does not enchantment to many people. To make it sweeter, blend with a few honey or water. Since they'll be to be had most effective in season from May to August, those end result may be tough to shop for in most supermarkets. You want to attempt getting prepared a tart cherry pie if you've had been given a few sweet cravings.

7.Sweet Potatoes

Sweet potatoes provide a wealthy deliver of fiber, nutrients B8, C, and A. Magnesium, a mineral that is pretty effective for sleep, is likewise widespread in candy potatoes. Magnesium has been tested to hurry up the way of falling asleep and enhance the extremely good of sleep.

There's a justification as to why a slice of pie crafted from candy potato or a massive Thanksgiving meal ought to probably make you nod off. These root veggies are generally low-glycemic carbohydrates that have been tested to useful resource in sleep, in evaluation to white potatoes and some one-of-a-type easy carbs.

Include this root vegetable for your regular rotation of supper aspects earlier than going to mattress. This adaptable vegetable pairs nicely with a substantial form of ingredients and may be organized in nearly any manner you pick out.

8.Prunes

Often called dried plums, prunes offer applicable vitamins to any type of food regimen. These dried culmination are a excellent source of healthy eating plan B6, magnesium, calcium, and amazing important vitamins that sell restful sleep. According to investigate, materials high in magnesium, together with prunes, can promote restful sleep and protect against sleep issues.

To gain from this fruit, eat a few piece of this fruit before sound asleep. If you don't like ingesting the dried form of this fruit, undergo in mind taking a plum as an opportunity.

9.Crackers and Cheese

Nearly on every occasion, this conventional kitchen staple and snack is nice. The scrumptious combination can also promote sleep. Owing to the presence of tryptophan, the famous amino acid that induces sleep, dairy products, collectively with cheese, milk, and yogurt, had been tested in severa research to beneficial aid with sleep.

While some research indicates that simple carbohydrates, at the side of crackers, impair sleep, distinct research indicates that they may honestly promote it. According to 1 research, excessive-glycemic index carbohydrates could possibly make you sleep greater quick than low-glycemic index carbohydrates.

Crackers and cheese are a bypass-to preference for a snack which you must eat before sleeping. Steer easy of heat cheeses which includes pepper jack and different notably spiced kinds. Try ingesting crackers produced with entire grains or vegetable flour if you'd want to stay a ways from white flour and smooth carbohydrates.

10. Kale

This lush, darkish inexperienced is probably your extraordinary superfood. Kale also consists of excessive tiers of magnesium and calcium, nutrients that useful aid sleep, in addition to nutrients K and C, fiber, and iron. A outstanding approach to growing your consumption of kale and taking component in greater sleep is to eat greater of it.

Kale want to be protected in severa recipes, inclusive of salads, however the fact that it has some bitterness via itself. Try munching chips crafted from this vegetable in case you're craving a few issue crunchy. These styles of chips can be bought already made or artificial at domestic.

eleven. Whole Grains

The blessings of entire grains for fitness are regularly stated. Whole grains encompass substances together with quinoa, rye, barley, and oats. Whole grains will beneficial resource in better sleep further to sporting fiber, iron, and antioxidants and reducing the attention of cholesterol and the risk of heart ailment. According to one 2020 research, postmenopausal ladies who fed on diets rich in those forms of components had a lot an awful lot less risk of sleeplessness.

Consume a plateful of oats (whole grain) in advance than going to mattress. Try growing a toast or sandwich the usage of sprouted grain bread for added complete grains.

12.Basil

This flavorful herb is an critical food for Italian recipes and a terrific accessory to almost any meal. Basil includes moderate sedative traits that would useful resource in sleep and reduce dyspepsia, that can also reason sleep disruption. According to an studies, basil nutritional supplements or beverages assisted a number of the studies individuals to sleep greater short and remain asleep longer. Consider taking basil tea or basil supplement in advance than drowsing.

thirteen.Carrots

Alpha-carotene, a crucial element in carrots, is vital for health and associated with stepped forward sleep. In the human frame, alpha-carotene is converted into food plan A. According to investigate from Pennsylvania University, normal alpha-carotene consumption advanced the first-rate of sleep. The studies moreover located that ingesting plans deficient in this nutrients made it difficult to fall asleep.

Drink a pitcher of carrot juice earlier than snoozing. Alternatively, you could need to nibble on a few humus with raw carrots.

14.Bananas

Banana is a well-known fruit essential in plenty of diets. Bananas, which may be rich in melatonin and potassium, assist the human body produce extra serotonin, which promotes sleep. Additionally, the wealthy magnesium awareness reduces cortisol stages, that could disturb sleep.

For extra nutrients, include a bit of crushed banana in a dish containing Greek yogurt. For greater protein, include peanut butter.

15.Honey

Honey is a sugary comfort meal that has a fantastic quantity of glucose content material cloth fabric and can help you sleep very rapid. It has been confirmed that honey prevents your frame from generating the wakefulness neurotransmitter orexin. A 2020 University of Saskatchewan studies located that ingesting raw honey extra suitable sleep nice.

According to this research, customers seeking out an herbal or natural sleep beneficial aid can utilize raw honey in choice to melatonin pills. Take a tablespoon of honey in advance than bedtime, or located a few in your cereal, toast, or tea.

16.Chamomile Tea

This is a traditional herbal treatment for sleeplessness. Chamomile, it's massive in herbal objects, is supported with the aid of generation. According to as a minimum one 2010 studies on the conventional plant, chamomile can assist with nausea, is a first-rate sleep resource, and includes anti inflammatory trends. Chamomiles are also packaged as vital oils or nutritional dietary dietary supplements similarly to tea.

Take a hot cup of chamomile tea in advance than sound asleep. Alternatively, you can prepare chamomile cookies and take them with your regular tea earlier than snoozing.

17.Tuna

The tuna fish is excessive in protein and is likewise a high-quality supply of minerals and nutrients. Also, it carries weight loss program B6 famously identified to promote sleep. Increasing your tuna consumption will help to procure this crucial weight loss program and enhance your sleep. Serotonin and melatonin are each produced with the assist of this food regimen.

Prepare crackers and tuna sandwiches or tuna salad on whole wheat bread and revel in them in advance than hitting the hay.

18.Lettuce

Do you experience tired from your facet salad? Although research display off the alternative, lettuce isn't normally considered one of the superior elements to promote sleep. The chemical lactucarium, positioned in lettuce, has herbal sedative trends that assist promote sleep and decrease anxiety. Lactucarium is found in all kinds of lettuce, with Romaine lettuce having the great stages of this biochemical.

Before going to sleep, prepare a sandwich with some Romaine lettuce. Make some lettuce tea in case you are incredibly bold and experimental.

19.Barley Powder

Green powders and smoothies often comprise barley powder, this is crafted from barley grass. Barley powder, which has been a long-acclaimed superfood, is concept to useful resource in sleep due to its tryptophan and food regimen B6 content material fabric. Barley grass's nutrients also can reduce disappointment and pressure. Prepare it in the midnight and each combo it proper right right into a smoothie or take it proper now before snoozing.

20.Shrimp

Shrimp, on the element of various shellfish inclusive of lobster, have fantastic portions of tryptophan, a nap-inducing amino acid. According to at least one studies, consuming seafood as a minimum one time each week added approximately progressed sleep and similarly cognitive regular general overall performance the following morning in each adults and youngsters. Eat seafood for supper or devour a shrimp cocktail as a snack earlier than looking at a few zzzs.

There are numerous food that can resource with sleep, further to nutrients, exercising, and pinnacle sleep conduct. Consult your fitness nutritionist or scientific physician to help determine the varieties of meals which is probably high-quality for you in advance than incorporating new devices into your diet plan or growing a new fitness routine.

Foods to Avoid Eating Before Sleeping

We all understand how crucial an brilliant night time time's sleep is. But did you recognize that what you eat in advance than bed should have an effect to your sleep amazing? There are effective foods that you want to avoid ingesting earlier than bedtime so that you can get the most from your close eye.

Here are some Foods to Avoid Eating Before Sleeping:

1.Spicy Foods:

Foods which might be immoderate in spice can motive indigestion and heartburn, that could make it difficult to fall asleep. If you're craving some element fantastically spiced, attempt to devour it earlier in the day simply so your frame has time to digest it in advance than bedtime. You're likely acquainted with the feeling of heartburn after consuming spicy meals. But did you recognize that quite spiced meals can also disrupt your sleep? It appears that there is a scientific reason inside the lower back of this. When you eat highly spiced food, your body temperature rises, and also you begin to sweat.

This increase in temperature can bring about confused sleep and hassle falling asleep. Additionally, capsaicin, the compound that offers chili peppers their warmth, can certainly boom frame temperature, making it more difficult to chill out and doze off. Finally, capsaicin additionally stimulates the discharge of adrenaline, which could make it hard to lighten up and go along with the go together with the flow off to sleep. In addition, especially spiced food can reason indigestion and acid reflux disorder disease sickness, every of that can keep you up at night. Avoid extensively spiced food in advance than bedtime in case you're seeking out an great night's sleep.

2.Caffeinated Foods and Drinks

Coffee, tea, energy drinks, and chocolate all encompass caffeine, that may be a stimulant which could make it tough to doze off. We've all been there - we are exhausted after an prolonged day, however we can not appear to doze off. So we advantage for a cup of espresso or a caffeinated soda, thinking that it's going to help us awaken enough to fall asleep. But then we lie in bed for hours, tossing and turning, because the caffeine keeps us extensive unsleeping.

Caffeine is a stimulant, and it without a doubt works through blocking certain receptors in the thoughts that would in any other case make us experience sleepy. In small doses, this will be useful if we want to live wide awake. But while we overdo it with caffeine, in particular close to bedtime, it is able to have the alternative effect and make it tough to go to sleep.

Caffeine blocks adenosine, a neurotransmitter that promotes sleepiness. As a quit end result, folks that consume caffeine past due in the day may also moreover moreover find it extra tough to fall asleep at night. In addition, caffeine can disrupt REM sleep, the inner most and most restful degree of sleep. As a end result, folks that eat caffeine may also awaken feeling groggy and unrested.

Cut lower returned for your consumption or keep away from it altogether within the middle of the night if you're your self finding lying conscious at night time time after having caffeine in advance in the day. That way, you will be more likely to get the restful sleep you need to experience your excellent at some point of the day. If you're craving something with caffeine, try to have it earlier in the day without a doubt so it might not have an impact to your sleep.

3.Fried Foods

We all comprehend that feeling: you're mendacity in bed, searching for to nod off, even as your belly begins growling. You tell yourself you could simply have a hint snack, and then you'll be able to sleep, but the next hassle you understand, you are standing in the front of the fridge, ingesting the whole lot in sight. Sounds familiar? If you find your self accomplishing for fried food past due at night, you're not on my own - however you'll be disrupting your sleep within the technique.

Fried factors are excessive in fat and energy, that could purpose indigestion and heartburn. And because of the reality they take longer to digest than distinctive styles of meals, they are capable of hold you feeling whole and prolonged through the night time. In addition, the immoderate-fat content material of fried meals can cause issues like sleep apnea, that can make it tough to get an brilliant night's relaxation. It is probably time to reduce on fried food. Your body - and your bed partner - will thank you for it! Foods which is probably excessive in fats and grease can purpose indigestion and heartburn, that might make it tough to go to sleep. If you're craving some thing fried, try and devour it in advance within the day just so your frame has time to digest it in advance than bedtime.

four.Acidic Foods

Acidic ingredients can have a disruptive effect on sleep. The acids in these meals can irritate the lining of the stomach, making it difficult to doze off and stay asleep. In addition, acidic ingredients can reason heartburn and indigestion, which also can make it tough to sleep. There are a few specific motives why acidic elements also can cause the ones troubles. First, acidic elements can stimulate the manufacturing of stomach acid.

This can cause heartburn and indigestion due to the truth the stomach acid isn't being nicely diluted with the aid of food. Second, acidic meals can worsen the liner of the stomach, inflicting soreness that makes it difficult to sleep. Third, acidic meals can reason infection in the gastrointestinal tract, which can also make contributions to sleep issues. While acidic food won't be the most effective purpose of sleep disruptions, they're capable of surely play a position in making it difficult to get an great night time's rest. Foods which is probably excessive in acid can motive heartburn and indigestion, that can make it tough to nod off. If you are craving some thing acidic, attempt to consume it earlier inside the day simply so your body has time to digest it earlier than bedtime.

five.Sugary Foods

Foods that are excessive in sugar can give you a sugar rush which can make it hard to doze off. We all recognize that sugary meals can supply us a short burst of strength, however did you understand that they can also disrupt our sleep? It's proper - at the same time as a sugar immoderate also can first of all appear to be the correct manner to electricity thru a past due-night time time have a examine session. Eventually, it'll come decrease once more to bite you.

The cause is that sugar influences our body's manufacturing of insulin, which in flip can result in an boom in adrenaline. And as every body apprehend, adrenaline is the hormone that facilitates us to stay alert and unsleeping. It's exceptional to persuade clean of sugary snacks earlier than bedtime if you're seeking to get an remarkable night time's sleep.

Chapter 11: What To Do To Get Better Sleep

Most human beings recognize that obtaining a amazing night time time's sleep is important for average fitness, but without a doubt achieving that intention can be tough. There are some simple subjects you can do, notwithstanding the fact that, to assist decorate your sleep great. First, putting in place a ordinary sleep agenda and sticking to it as plenty as feasible is one way to move. Going to bed and waking up at the same time each day permits to adjust your frame's herbal sleep rhythm.

Secondly, you may want to create a calming bedtime everyday to assist sign on your frame that it's time to wind down for the night time time. This may additionally additionally embody taking a heat bathtub or reading a ebook earlier than bed. Also, ensuring that your snoozing surroundings is snug and dark can get you suitable sleep - every too much light and an excessive amount of noise can interfere with sleep. In the sections beneath, we'll delve into this properly so you have to make an knowledgeable choice and the manner and why you need to get better sleep.

Design a Sleep Schedule That You Can Easily Follow Through With

We all understand that feeling of being exhausted after an prolonged day. Whether we were running difficult at the administrative center or chasing after children all day, once in a while all we need to do is crash into mattress and preference for an awesome night time time's sleep. But did you recognize that there can be this sort of component as a top notch sleep time table? And following it could be vital to your health and properly-being.

There are truly specific sorts of sleep schedules: monophasic and polyphasic. Monophasic sleep is while you sleep for one long stretch in the course of the night time time, whilst polyphasic sleep is while you cut up your sleep into numerous shorter durations within the direction of the day or night. Most human beings are monophasic sleepers, however there are a few who swear through polyphasic sleep (which incorporates well-known historic figures like Leonardo da Vinci and Benjamin Franklin).

There are experts and cons to each kinds of sleep schedules. Monophasic sleep is the maximum not unusual and considered the herbal way to sleep, however it is able to be hard to paste to if you have a hectic way of life. Polyphasic sleep may be extra handy and will will let you get greater achieved in an afternoon, however it could additionally be disruptive in your natural body clock (not to say socially awkward in case you're attempting to find to take a nap within the center of the day!).

Ultimately, it's miles vital to find what works first-rate for you. If you're struggling to get enough relaxation at night time time time, test with awesome kinds of sound asleep patterns till you find one which allows you revel in nicely-rested and energized inside the path of the day. Your frame will thanks!

Pay a Great Deal of Attention to What You Eat

When it includes getting an first rate night time time's sleep, most people consciousness on growing the right mattress room environment. But the fact is, what you eat may want to have in reality as massive of an impact on your sleep exquisite as how darkish and quiet your room is. That's due to the fact the substances you eat could have an impact at the hormones that adjust sleep, together with melatonin and serotonin.

Eating a nutritious weight loss plan with masses of stop result, vegetables, and whole grains can assist sell healthy sleep styles. And heading off substances which is probably excessive in sugar and sensitive carbs can help save you spikes in blood sugar that could disrupt sleep. Pay hobby to what you consume can be the critical problem to in the long run getting a few rest.

Create a Conducive Environment for Sleep

Most folks have had the experience of tossing and turning all night time time time, unable to get a single wink of sleep. It may be disturbing, specially when you have to evoke early for paintings or college day after today. There are some matters you can do to help yourself sleep better, even though. One is to create a conducive surroundings for sleep. This manner ensuring your bed room is cool, darkish, and quiet. You may additionally additionally bear in mind making an investment in a cushty mattress and bedding.

Creating an surroundings that promotes rest will assist your body to wind down at night time and put together for sleep. In addition, putting in place a normal sleep time table additionally may be beneficial. If you visit mattress and wake up at the same time every day, your frame will start to expect it and may be more likely to doze off fast even as it's time to show it in for the night. If you are having trouble napping, attempt growing a more conducive surroundings and stay with a ordinary sleep time table. With a touch effort, you have got as a way to get the restful night time's sleep you need.

Reduce How Much You Sleep within the Afternoon

What's the excellent manner to get an exquisite night time time's sleep? Many people may additionally want to say that it's miles all approximately getting enough close to-eye. However, research indicates that the tremendous of your sleep is just as crucial as the amount. One manner to assist make certain that you're getting awesome sleep is to restrict your afternoon naps.

It may also additionally seem counterintuitive, but snoozing inside the afternoon can in truth make it greater hard to go to sleep at night. That's because of the fact dozing can lessen your middle of the night sleep stress, making it more tough to get an entire eight hours of near-eye. In addition, snoozing can purpose fragmented sleep, this is even as you awaken regularly at some stage in the night time.

If you're seeking out a way to decorate the fine of your sleep, restricting your afternoon naps is a awesome area to begin. By doing so, you will be much more likely to feel rested and refreshed when you awaken inside the morning.

Worry Less

We all understand the sensation of tossing and turning at night time time, our minds racing as we fear about everything it genuinely is on our plate. But what you couldn't understand is that worrying can sincerely have a sizable effect for your sleep. Whether it's far a large venture at art work, a looming reduce-off date, or a fight with a friend, stress can take a toll on our sleep. In reality, traumatic is one of the most not unusual causes of insomnia. When we worry, our our our bodies pass into "fight or flight" mode, releasing pressure hormones like cortisol.

This ought to make it tough to doze off and stay asleep, as our our bodies have become ready for motion in place of rest. In addition, disturbing can result in racing thoughts and a mean feeling of unease, making it hard to lighten up enough to doze off. Fortunately, there are a few clean topics you can do to assist harm the priority cycle and get a better night time time's sleep.

First, attempt to designate a particular time every day to worry. This will can help you limit your stressful to a attainable period, in preference to letting it take over your entire day (and night time). Second, exercise a few relaxation strategies in advance than bedtimes, which incorporates deep respiration or present day muscle relaxation.

This can assist to calm your body and thoughts, making it less complicated to float off to sleep. Finally, go through in thoughts that now not all issues are really worth losing sleep over. If you find your self disturbing about some component that appears minor or now not going to occur, try and allow it skip and popularity on getting some rest. By taking those steps, you could help yourself smash the cycle of worry and get the restful sleep you want.

Dim the Lights

Why is it that after we're looking for to sleep, our thoughts involves a choice that it is time to think about the entirety we want to do tomorrow? For most human beings, it's miles simplest a truth of existence. But there may be a manner to assist our brains loosen up earlier than mattress: through dimming the lights. According to analyze, exposure to vibrant mild in the night can intervene with our natural sleep cycle.

Our our bodies are designed to comply with the natural cycle of daylight hours and darkness, and at the same time as we disclose ourselves to bright light in the nighttime, it is able to ship symptoms that it's miles but time to be extensive conscious and alert. Dimming the lighting signals to our our our bodies that it is time to begin generating melatonin, the hormone that makes us sense sleepy. Also, dimming the lighting can help sign to our brains that it is time to wind down for the night time. Try turning down the lighting in your mattress room a few hours earlier than you go to bed. You may also clearly find out that it makes it a great deal less hard to glide off.

Hush the Noises

When it is time to hit the hay, maximum people want whole silence that allows you to float off right right right into a deep sleep. But because it appears, a few mild facts noise can absolutely be useful in engaging in a top notch night time time's rest. Whether it's far the sound of raindrops or the hum of a fan, so-referred to as "white noise" can assist to masks disruptive noises that might otherwise keep you up at night time time.

Whether it is the sound of traffic out of doors your window or your roommate's TV within the next room, extra noise ought to make it tough to nod off and live asleep. That's why many human beings find it beneficial to create a "hush" environment earlier than bed. By turning off electronics, closing the blinds, and the use of a white noise tool, you may create a space this is freed from distractions and better conducive to sleep. In addition, hushing noises can assist to masks undesirable sounds from out of doors, making it less tough to go with the flow off right right right into a peaceful close eye.

In addition, white noise can assist to lessen the general degree of data noise to your environment, making it much less difficult to loosen up and nod off. Try putting in region a white noise tool in advance than hitting the pillow. It definitely would probably help you go along with the glide off into a non violent close eye.

Create a Pre-Bed Routine

You know the sensation. You've had a long day, and you're in the long run prepared to hit the hay, however your mind is racing, and you cannot seem to lighten up. If this sounds familiar, it is probably time to create a pre-mattress ordinary. A pre-mattress regular can help cue your body that it's time to wind down for the night time. This may include some thing as easy as taking a couple of minutes to test or stretching earlier than you get in bed. By growing a constant ritual in advance than sleep, you may train your frame to begin feeling sleepy on the identical time every night time time time. And whilst you ultimately do waft off to sleep, you'll be more likely to live asleep because you may no longer be tossing and turning all night. Try growing a pre-bed ordinary and be conscious if it makes a difference. Sweet dreams!

Play Low-Volume Soothing Sounds

We all recognize how important an awesome night time's sleep is. But every so often, it could be tough to get our minds to sluggish down sufficient certainly to doze off. That's wherein soothing sounds can are to be had available. Listening to calming, amusing song or nature sounds can help to gradual your coronary heart price and respiratory and ease you right into a restful country.

In addition, the mild, rhythmic styles of these sounds can assist to lull you into sleep. And if you awaken inside the midnight, the sounds can offer a relaxing ancient beyond noise that can help you drift backtrack to sleep. Try gambling a few soothing sounds earlier than you switch it in. You may in reality discover your self sleeping higher than ever in advance than.

Declutter Your Bedroom

A cluttered mattress room can be a breeding ground for dust mites, mildew, and mold - all of that would reason allergic reactions and function an impact on sleep amazing. In fact, research has proven that people with muddle of their bedrooms have a tendency to have extra hassle falling asleep and are more likely to experience sunlight hours fatigue. Similar studies have validated that human beings sleep better in a tidy and prepared place.

When your bed room is whole of litter, it can be tough to lighten up.

Your thoughts may be racing with all of the assets you need to do, which makes it difficult to go with the flow off to sleep. But at the equal time as your bed room is straightforward and serene, it is a terrific deal simpler to loosen up and nod off. By decluttering your bed room, you could create a calmer, greater inviting location that promotes higher sleep. Plus, you could moreover experience the delivered benefit of being able to discover matters extra without problems even as you need them! Decluttering your mattress room is a fantastic area to begin.

Choose a Comfy Bedding

Everyone merits an wonderful night time's sleep. But among paintings, circle of relatives, and social duties, it may be hard to get the advocated seven to 8 hours a night time. One manner to improve your sleep is to spend money on comfortable bedding. A comfortable mattress and pillow are important, of direction.

But don't forget approximately the sheets! Soft, exceptional sheets could make all the difference in how nicely you sleep. After all, there is not anything worse than tossing and turning all night time time time because of the reality your sheets are scratchy or too hot. And in case you have a tendency to get cold at night, flannel sheets are a tremendous opportunity.

They're comfy and warm, but they're additionally breathable, so that you won't get too heat. A supportive bed and pillow can help lessen tossing and turning, and breathable sheets can maintain you from getting too warm or too cold during the night.

In addition, selecting bedding that fits your snoozing fashion can also make a distinction. For example, detail sleepers regularly find that softer pillows offer the best useful useful resource for their neck and shoulders. By taking the time to choose the proper bedding,

176

you can revel in a greater restful night time time's sleep.

Use a Great Pillow

Have you ever woken up with a crick in your neck or decided your self tossing and turning all night time prolonged? If so, then it is probably time to rethink your pillow. Most humans do not count on instances approximately their pillows, but they will truely make a big distinction in your high-quality of sleep. If you are waking up with a neckache or stiffness, it is possibly time to put money into a new pillow.

There are lots of things to don't forget while selecting a pillow, at the side of firmness, filling, and duration. You want to additionally reflect onconsideration on your sleep position and whether or not or now not you commonly usually tend to sweat at night. Choosing the proper pillow ought to make a world of distinction in terms of having a awesome night time's sleep. For instance, aspect sleepers need a pillow this is company and supportive, at the equal time as belly sleepers need a thinner and softer pillow.

Pillows are also to be had in numerous substances, from down feathers to reminiscence foam. Experimenting with precise pillows allow you to discover the proper one for you. And when you find out the right pillow, you'll be amazed at how lots higher you sleep.

With such plenty of alternatives available, it can be formidable to find the exceptional pillow. But taking the time to find the right you'll in reality repay in terms of higher sleep. A superb night time time's sleep is crucial for standard fitness and nicely-being, so it's far virtually well worth taking the time to find out the quality pillow.

Show Some Gratitude

Picture this: It's 11 PM, and you're tossing and handing over bed, looking to doze off. But no matter how tough you try, your thoughts may not close off. You start thinking about all the subjects you need to do tomorrow, and earlier than you understand it, it's far morning. Sound acquainted? If you have ever struggled with insomnia, you're now not by myself. In reality, steady with the National Sleep Foundation, one in 3 human beings have difficulty falling asleep or staying asleep at least once every week.

Luckily, there are various of things you could do to enhance your sleep top notch - one in each of it clearly is displaying gratitude. One purpose for that is that gratitude permits to lessen pressure and tension. When we are grateful for the great things in our lives, it lets in us to allow bypass of the worries and issues that might hold us up at night time time time. Gratitude moreover promotes feelings of happiness and contentment, which can be soothing and calming in advance than bed.

Expressing gratitude has been proven to decrease stress ranges and improve temper, both of which might be critical for falling asleep. When you feel stressed or stressful, your body produces cortisol, a hormone that makes it greater hard to nod off. By assessment, gratitude allows to lessen cortisol stages and sell the manufacturing of serotonin - a chemical that plays an essential role in regulating sleep.

Additionally, gratitude can help to boom emotions of average nicely-being and satisfaction with lifestyles - more key additives for a great night time time's rest. Try expressing gratitude in advance than bedtime. It just may likely help you finally get the relaxation you need!

Practice Yoga

Yoga is a shape of contemplative exercise that consists of mindfulness, awareness, and health. The machine dates returned more than 3 thousand years and is based totally mostly on Indian philosophy. Nevertheless, there are numerous yoga faculties and variations. Each version stresses special sports activities activities or postures, respiration strategies, and meditation sports.

Yoga can revel in quite a few useful effects on nicely-being, which include improving one's emotional and mental properly-being and reducing strain, easing a few kinds of pain, losing weight, and getting a higher night time's sleep.

More than 80-5 percentage of yoga observers record a whole lot a lot less pressure, and further than fifty-5 percentage document better sleep. Numerous research show that yoga can decorate sleep for pretty a few people. As more sleep is not constantly correlated with better sleep and preferred properly being, those investigations normally location extra emphasis on sleep awesome than its quantity. While each sleeper has their very personal interpretation of what quality sleep way, maximum agree that it consists of feeling rested and unbothered day after today.

Use Lavender and Chamomile

Scent has a effective impact on the thoughts. Certain smells can trigger reminiscences and emotions, whilst others have to have a chilled effect. For centuries, lavender and chamomile were used to sell rest and higher sleep. The scent of these herbs can assist to sluggish down the activity of the disturbing tool, making it simpler to nod off. For some humans, it's far strain or tension that keeps them up. For others, it is a chronic ache or a few other medical state of affairs. Whatever the cause, insomnia can be a annoying and debilitating hassle.

Luckily, there are some natural remedies which could help. Both lavender and chamomile are widely recognized for their calming houses, and they'll be very effective in selling sleep. In addition, each lavender and chamomile encompass compounds that have a sedative effect on the body. When used before mattress, those herbs can assist to enhance sleep exceptional and duration. As a end result, lavender and chamomile are often encouraged for those who struggle with insomnia or other sleep troubles.

Lavender oil may be delivered to a diffuser or utilized in a bedtime rub down, on the identical time as chamomile tea is a well-known bedtime beverage. In addition to their calming outcomes, each lavender and chamomile moreover have moderate sedative homes, that can further help to sell sleep. Give those herbal remedies a try, and you may now not remorse what you probable did.

Sleep Hygiene

Changing our carrying activities is probably all it takes to create advanced sleep conditions. Our our our our bodies are designed to loosen up often, now not to live pumped up before falling asleep proper away. That is why there is a need for extraordinary sleep hygiene.

 The name "sleep hygiene" is on occasion a bit perplexing because it does not embody cleaning one's tooth or washing one's face earlier than bed. (But undergo in thoughts to moreover accomplish the ones subjects!)

Science-based totally completely simply sports referred to as "sleep hygiene" can play a crucial characteristic among a confused night time and a non violent one through supporting to create the proper conditions for healthy sleep before bed and in some unspecified time within the future of the day.

Hold, Let Go, And Then Restart Yourself

Take some time to unwind and make your thoughts and frame extra at peace so that you can also moreover enjoy tons greater inside the period in-between and greater able to appreciating what takes vicinity next.

Start Meditation

Try Reset: Relax Your Mind and Body for Ten minutes.

What Are The Telltale Indications Of Bad Sleeping Habits?

www.ingramcontent.com/pod-product-compliance
Lightning Source LLC
Chambersburg PA
CBHW060223030426
42335CB00014B/1324